Reviews of *The Infection Game – Life is an*

GW00643746

Throughout our years of training as doctors we were told ... would find infections as the root cause of many common inflammatory diseases afflicting mankind. Today, current scientific evidence has corroborated this hypothesis in many conditions as research has shown associations between infections and conditions such as inflammatory bowel disease, arthritis, Alzheimer's, chronic fatigue syndrome and cardiovascular disease to name a few. We now experience such epidemics ubiquitously. Furthermore, the Deputy Chief Medical Officer for England, who has special expertise in, and responsibility for, pandemics, tells us that the next most likely plague to affect humanity is the H7N9 strain of the flu virus which is circulating in poultry in China with a potential 38% mortality rate.

Dr Myhill's new book is an eloquent and informative text which explores the relationship between infections and various medical conditions. She offers a wealth of accessible information whether you are interested in strengthening your immune system to combat epidemics or benefiting from the simple, safe, scientific techniques she describes for preventing chronic disease. Dr Myhill's book may well make the difference between succumbing to infections or having sufficient resistance and resilience to withstand their onslaught.

Dr Shideh Pouria, MB BS BSc MRCP(UK) PhD, Consultant Physician

I run a laboratory specialising in the diagnosis of chronic infection. We know for a fact that chronic infection is a major root cause of chronic fatigue, inflammation, degenerative disease, neurological disease and cancer. In this book, Dr Myhill astutely identifies the big issues and, more importantly, what we can all do to prevent and treat infection. In her usual straightforward, pragmatic style she details regimes that are highly effective but within the power of us all to put in place. If you are to stand a chance of surviving the next epidemic and living to your full potential you must read this book, absorb it and… just do it!

Dr Armin Schwarzbach, Armin Labs, Germany

In her inimitable fashion, Dr Myhill once again makes a plain and straightforward case for improving our health and longevity with the natural tools we all have access to: a good paleo-keto diet, adequate nutrition and natural antimicrobial remedies. Engaging and accessible to all, this book needs to be at the top of everyone's first aid kit.

Dr Sarah Davies, MB ChB MRCGP AFMCP2015,
General Practitioner, Stockport, UK

Dedication

SM: 'To my lovely patients, who have been willing guinea pigs and most forgiving when my suggestions have not worked. However, in doing so, they have pushed forward the frontiers of practical medicine.'

CR: 'For Kathryn – I met Kathryn on Facebook in 2010 and we have grown to be the best of friends, running Dr Myhill's groups online since 2012. Not only has Kathryn survived extreme adversity, but she now embraces life and faces all the many challenges of a chronic illness head-on, always with a smile on her face. She has fallen in love with Mark, a man who sees her inner strength – their story is a living example of *amor vincit omnia.*'

The Infection Game
Life is an arms race

Dr Sarah Myhill MB BS
&
Craig Robinson MA (Oxon)

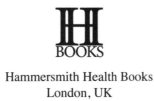

Hammersmith Health Books
London, UK

First published in 2018 by Hammersmith Health Books – an imprint of
Hammersmith Books Limited
4/4A Bloomsbury Square, London WC1A 2RP, UK
www.hammersmithbooks.co.uk

The information contained in this book is for educational purposes only. It is
the result of the study and the experience of the authors. Whilst the information
and advice offered are believed to be true and accurate at the time of going to
press, neither the authors nor the publisher can accept any legal responsibility or
liability for any errors or omissions that may have been made or for any adverse
effects which may occur as a result of following the recommendations given
herein. Always consult a qualified medical practitioner if you have any concerns
regarding your health.

British Library Cataloguing in Publication Data: A CIP record of this book is
available from the British Library.

Print ISBN 978-1-78161-142-5
Ebook ISBN 978-1-78161-143-2

Commissioning editor: Georgina Bentliff
Designed and typeset by: Julie Bennett, Bespoke Publishing Ltd
Cover design by: Julie Bennett, Bespoke Publishing Ltd
Cover photograph: Shutterstock/MaleWitch
Index: Dr Laurence Errington
Production: Helen Whitehorn, Pathprojects Ltd
Printed and bound by: TJ International Ltd, UK

Contents

Contents

Acknowledgements

We would like to thank the following sources for permission to quote their words in this book:

- For quotations from *Blackadder Goes Forth* and *Blackadder Back & Forth* in Chapters 4 and 18, United Agents (www.unitedagents.co.uk)
- For the quotation from *PERELANDRA* by CS Lewis © copyright CS Lewis Pte Ltd 1944, in chapter 7, Rachel Churchill
- For the quotation from Dr Marik in Chapter 9, Dr Marik himself (marikpe@evms.edu)
- For the many quotations from *Vaccination Policy and the UK Government: The Untold Truth* in Chapter 14, the authors Christina England and Lucija Tomljenovic PhD
- For the quotation in Chapter 28 from Dr Burakgazi AZ, Neuroscience Section, Department of Medicine, Virginia Tech Carilion School of Medicine, Roanoke, VA, USA from the *International Journal of Neuroscience* 2014; 124 (11). www.tandfonline.com/doi/abs/10.3109/00207454.2013.879582, which is reprinted by permission of Taylor & Francis Ltd, www.tandfonline.com

About the Authors

Dr Sarah Myhill MB BS, qualified in medicine (with Honours) from
Middlesex Hospital Medical School in 1981 and has since focused tirelessly on
identifying and treating the underlying causes of health problems, especially the
'diseases of civilisation' with which we are beset in the West. She has worked in the
NHS and private practice and for 17 years was the Hon. Secretary of the British Society
for Ecological Medicine, which focuses on the causes of disease and treating through
diet, supplements and avoiding toxic stress. She helps to run, and lectures at, the
Society's training courses and also lectures regularly on organophosphate poisoning, the
problems of silicone, and chronic fatigue syndrome.
Visit her website at www.drmyhill.co.uk

Craig Robinson MA, took a first in Mathematics at Oxford University in
1985. He then joined Price Waterhouse and qualified as a Chartered Accountant in 1988,
after which he worked as a lecturer in the private sector, and also in the City of London,
primarily in Financial Sector Regulation roles. Craig first met Sarah in 2001, as a patient
for the treatment of his CFS, and since then they have developed a professional working
relationship, where he helps with the maintenance of www.drmyhill.co.uk, the
moderating of Dr Myhill's Facebook groups and other ad hoc projects, as well as with
the editing and writing of her books.

Introduction

The hypothesis – disease, degeneration and death are all driven by infection.

A mathematical proof, like a chess problem, to be aesthetically satisfying must possess three qualities: inevitability, unexpectedness and economy.
A Mathematician's Apology 1940 Godfrey Harold Hardy (1887 – 1947)

Inevitability: We will all die. My job as a doctor is both to postpone that moment for as long as possible and also to maximise quality of life – quantity and quality.

Unexpectedness: We have been led to believe that infection is a killer of the past. Wrong. We now know our big killers, from cancers and coronaries to dementia and diabetes, are largely driven by infection. Slow-burn herpes viruses, once acquired, live in our bodies for life to create immunological havoc. Microbes in the fermenting gut drive gut tumours. They also drive psychiatric disease and arthritis. Neurological disease is the commonest cause of death in Westerners and all varieties have an infectious driver. Indeed, it is difficult to find a pathology (illness) that does not have an infectious associate.

Economy: The solutions are intellectually simple but practically difficult. Cheap and effective defences are within the grasp of us all. We have all the weapons we need. What follows in this book provides the intellectual imperative and practical know-how to conquer the established, prevent the potential and postpone the inevitable.

This book, then, possesses the three qualities of a mathematical proof to our hypothesis. However, life is not a single chess problem but rather a succession of different problems, a *game* of chess – in the black corner we have our clever, manipulative and determined opponents which range from the rhinovirus pawns of the common cold and the nasty knights of neisseria, to the *Borrelia* bishops and the rotten rooks of retrovirus. In the white corner we have our standing army to defend the middle ground of disease. We have our paleo-pawns that form the front line, our vitamin C castles and our herbal knights in shining armour; our iodine purple-robed bishops and our antibiotic queens. It really is a case of War and Peace.

Read on. Use your brain. Just do it.

Stylistic note: Use of the first person singular in this book refers to me, Dr Myhill. One can assume that the medicine and biochemistry are mine, as edited by Craig Robinson, and that the classical and mathematical references are Craig's.

Part I

Life is an arms race that we are already losing

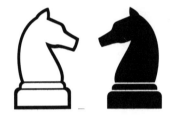

Chapter 1

Life is an arms race

There ain't no such thing as a free lunch.*
Or maybe there is…

You and I are a free lunch for bacteria, yeasts, viruses, fleas, flies, ticks, worms and… what else? These invaders have been struggling for survival for all the many billions of years during which we have been evolving. Their struggle has always had the ultimate aim of making themselves at home in our very comfortable bodies. They have developed extraordinary and complex strategies to succeed. In response, we have evolved defences, including a fantastic immune system which is just as intelligent and adaptive as these invaders. Indeed, the immune system shares many attributes with the brain – it is intelligent, decision making and just as mysterious.

We currently think we have won this arms race, but we are wrong. We have been lulled into a false sense of security by drugs and vaccinations. We are in the 'phoney war' – the enemy is evolving fast and is just over the horizon. Resistance to antimicrobials is already a major cause of death and the efficacy of vaccination has been over-egged. We need a fresh approach to the arms race.

Footnote: This phrase is thought to have derived from the 19th-century practice in American bars of offering a free lunch to entice in drinking customers. Robert Heinlein's 1966 novel, *The Moon Is a Harsh Mistress*, brought the phrase into common usage.

The threat of antibiotic resistance [to mankind] is much more serious than global warming.

Dame Sally Claire Davies, DBE FMEDSCI FRS,
Chief Medical Officer for England (1949 –)

We need a new antibiotic to be developed every 15 years for eternity to control new infections.

Professor Jeremy Nicholson,
Medical Director of the MRC NHR National Phenome Centre

Historical note – The 'Phoney War' (German: *'Sitzkrieg'*) was an eight-month period at the start of World War II during which there were no major military land operations on the Western Front. It began in September 1939 and ended with the German *Blitzkrieg* attack on France and the Low Countries in May 1940. We must not forget that the *Sitzkrieg* ended with the *Blitzkrieg*. We should prepare for our own personal *Blitzkriegs*.

Of course, as a doctor, patients do not visit me when they are well. They come with diseases. My special interest has been treating people with chronic fatigue syndrome (CFS). Pure CFS results from poor energy delivery mechanisms. Myalgic encephalitis (ME) results when the fatigue is accompanied by inflammation. I now know that this inflammation is often driven by microbes, such as herpes viruses (especially Epstein Barr virus), *Borrelia* (Lyme), *Bartonella*, *Babesia*, *Mycoplasma*, *Rickettsia*, *Yersinia* and many others. What is so fascinating is that these microbes have co-existed with and evolved alongside our ancestors for millions of years. The fact that they are starting to cause infections *now* is symptomatic of our declining ability to resist them. This is a direct result of modern Western diets and lifestyles. We are already losing the arms race. The *Sitzkrieg* is nearly over and the *Blitzkrieg* will soon be upon us.

So, when people come to me with their ME (remember ME implies inflammation, which in turn often implies infection), it is not sufficient for me simply to tackle the particular microbe that is suspect or has been identified. I must take a holistic view. Indeed, if people with ME (PwME) have one microbe on board, then it is highly likely that they will have others on board too, for the very same reasons that they have the one that is suspected or has been identified. This means my job must have at least a two-pronged approach.

- First, I must teach people a general approach to avoiding and treating infection and start to get them ahead of the game with their own personal arms race. Here I am being a 'doctor' in the proper sense of the word – doctor is an 'agentive' noun of the Latin verb *docēre* meaning 'to teach'.

- Secondly, I need to put in place effective strategies that will tackle the particular microbe or microbes that have successfully made themselves at home in the PwME's comfortable body and are making life a misery in the process. The misery results from fatigue (because the immune system is using up all available energy) and inflammation (which results in every chronic symptom the body can experience).

Even if you do not suffer from CFS/ME, the above interventions are important for two further reasons:

1. Most chronic diseases, as detailed in Chapter 2, are driven by infection.

2. As a species, we are heading for disaster. Declining immunity puts us at risk of death with the next epidemic. Indeed, throughout evolution more people have died as a result of infection than any other cause. Most recently, the Spanish 'flu (H1N1) epidemic at the end of World War 1 killed an estimated 50-100 million people.

Historical note: For those who are interested please see *Influenza: The Once and Future Pandemic* by Jeffery K Taubenberger, MD PhD, and David M Morens, MD[1] which looks at the 1918 pandemic in detail, with reference to possible future pandemics.

The interventions I ask people to make are difficult. Understanding the how and the why is empowering and gives us the necessary determination to make these changes.

Knowledge is Power.

Sir Francis Bacon, *Meditationes Sacrae* (1597)
(22 January 1561 – 9 April 1626)

The exact quotation is 'for knowledge itself is a power whereby he knoweth' which is even more apposite here – not only do we need to have the knowledge but we also need the wisdom to apply that knowledge.

Chapter 2

Infections that drive modern Western diseases

We all love it, especially me, when single infections cause singular diseases with specific symptoms that resolve with an antibiotic. These conditions make me look like a magician and feel like a god! The patients are awfully grateful too. But life is no longer that easy – microbes are sneaking in at the back door aided by modern junk food and unhealthy lifestyles.

> *'Cherchez la femme,'* said Alexandre Dumas in the 1854 novel *The Mohicans of Paris*, implying that no matter what the problem, a woman was at the root cause. (Alexandre Dumas (24 July 1802 – 5 December 1870), also known as 'Alexandre Dumas, *père*', was a French writer most famous nowadays for writing *The Three Musketeers*.) We now know better. It should have been *'Cherchez l'homme'* – but I digress and my editor is a man who has nonetheless had the title of honorary woman bestowed upon him! In the case of chronic modern illnesses, we should say: *'Cherchez les microbes, les sucres, la junk food, les pesticides, les métaux lourds et la vie moderne!'*

We now recognise that the potentially lethal conditions listed in Table 2.1 have the infectious associations shown in the right hand column (see next page).

Table 2.1: Infectious agents associated with serious conditions

Disease	Associated microbes and infections	Mechanisms	Other causal associations
Dementia: this is now the commonest cause of death in Westerners.[2]	*Borrelia* (Lyme disease) *Toxoplasma* Herpes virus 1 (cold sores) Herpes virus 2 (genital herpes) Herpes viruses 6 and 7 Cytomegalovirus *Cryptococcus* Cystercercosis *Mycoplasma* Syphilis HIV Creutzfeld Jacob disease (CJD) (the infectious particle is uncertain) Possibly *Helicobacter pylori* and *Chlamydia pneumoniae* Fungal infection	There is a cumulative effect – the greater the infectious burden and the greater the antibody response to that, then the greater the inflammation and risk of dementia. I suspect 'prion' protein is the biofilm (i.e. the shield) that defends microbes from our immune system. Non-REM sleep clears this protein (amyloid) from the brain (see Chapter 6 (page 41).	Sugar (sugar feeds microbes) and refined carbohydrates. Dementia is also known as 'type 3 diabetes'. The ketogenic diet can reverse dementia.[3] Dr Dale Bredesen used a ketogenic diet and supplements to reverse cognitive decline in Alzheimer's patients. Lack of deep, non-REM sleep is not just a risk factor but also a predictor of Alzheimer's. Heavy metals and pesticides damage the immune system. Arterial disease – this is also driven by sugar and other infections.
Arterial disease	Oral infection (gram negative bacteria), especially gum disease Herpes viruses *Helicobacter pylori* *Chlamydia pneumoniae* Cytomegalovirus *Bartonella* *Yersinia*	Arterial disease impairs blood supply, resulting in heart disease, dementia and organ failure	Sugar is also a risk factor – again sugar feeds microbes. Microbes in the mouth easily get into the bloodstream. Simple chewing can result in bacteraemia (bacteria in the blood).
Cancer: 20% of all cancers have a single infectious associate; others are multifactorial.[4]	*Helicobacter pylori* Epstein Barr virus Human papilloma virus Hepatitis B Hepatitis C	Infections drive inflammation, which drives cancer	Diabetes (ergo sugar) doubles the risk of cancer of the colon, rectum, breast, womb, kidney, bladder, liver, pancreas, lymphoma and probably others. (See also our book *Prevent and Cure Diabetes* for a more detailed analysis.)

Stomach cancer	Abnormal gut microbiome, including *Helicobacter pylori* Anaerobic bacteria	As above	Vitamin C kills microbes in the upper gut and so prevents the fermentation of nitrates to nitrites and nitrosamines
Oesophageal cancer: now the fastest increasing cancer in Westerners	Human papilloma virus My guess is also microbes from the upper fermenting gut	As above	Sugar, smoking and alcohol are also risk factors
Colon cancer	Abnormal gut flora resulting from Western diets *Streptococcus bovis* Schistosomiasis	I suspect, abnormal fermentation products	Paleo-ketogenic diets and vitamin C are highly protective
Oral cancer	Gum disease		Smoking and alcohol are also risk factors
Gall bladder cancer	*Salmonella typhi* Liver flukes		
Cervical cancer	Human papilloma virus		The contraceptive pill and smoking further increase the risk
Lung cancer	*Chlamydia pneumoniae* HIV		Smoking accounts for 75% of cases Air pollution accounts for most others Sugar and refined carbohydrates are risk factors
Bladder and kidney tumours	HTLV1 (see page 10) In Africa, bladder cancers are largely caused by the parasite *Schistosoma* that leads to schistosomiasis	Chronic inflammation due to bacterial translocation …	… that is, microbes which spill over from the fermenting gut and are excreted in urine are a risk factor Smoking Pesticides[5]

9

Disease	Associated microbes and infections	Mechanisms	Other causal associations
Lymphomas	Retrovirus e.g. HTLV1 (human leukaemia T cell virus type) Epstein Barr virus HIV	Viruses hijack the cell's normal mechanisms for replication	Toxic chemicals, especially pesticides
Leukaemia	HTLV1	Ditto above	Ditto above
Skin cancer	Beta papilloma virus		
Mesothelioma	SV40 (simian vacuolating virus 40 or simian virus 40, a polyomavirus found in both monkeys and humans) from vaccination (many vaccines are now contaminated with SV40) plus asbestos exposure		
Prostate cancer	Retrovirus, e.g. XMRV		
Breast cancer	Retrovirus HERV		Contraceptive pill and HRT are risk factors
Vascular tumours	*Bartonella*		
Brain tumours	Human polyoxoma virus		
Kaposi's sarcoma	Human herpes virus 8 (HHV8)		Becomes apparent with the immune-suppression of AIDs

The following chronic degenerative conditions also have infectious associations:

Table 2.2: Infectious agents associated with chronic degenerative conditions

Disease	Associated microbes ind infections	Possible mechanisms	Other associations
Myalgic encephalitis (ME)	All herpes viruses, especially Epstein Barr virus *Borrelia* (Lyme), *Bartonella* and *Babesia* *Mycoplasma*	The low grade immune activity punches an immunological hole in the energy bucket	See our book, *Diagnosis and Treatment of CFS and ME – it's mitochondria, not hypochondria* 2nd Edition for a more detailed analysis
Osteoarthritis and connective tissue disease	Most cases are due to allergy to foods and/ or microbes from the fermenting gut	These easily spill over into the bloodstream with the potential to drive inflammatory reactions at other sites (e.g. joints). This is called bacterial translocation	Arthritis is part of metabolic syndrome. See our book *Prevent and Cure Diabetes – delicious diets not dangerous drugs* for a more detailed analysis
Acne *Proprionibacterium acnes*	Ditto above	Ditto above	
Inflammatory arthritis	Ankylosing spondylitis is associated with *Klebsiella* Rheumatoid arthritis is associated with *Proteus mirablis*, rubella virus *Bartonella* *Yersinia*	This is not acute infection but an inflammatory process driven by infection. Some cases respond well to antibiotics	Most cases respond well to the paleo-ketogenic (PK) diet (see page 234 and our book, *The PK Cookbook*) and vitamin C to bowel tolerance (see Chapter 9, page 55). (The PK diet is very low in carbs and high in saturated fat and fibre so the body can run on fatty acids rather than glucose.)

Disease	Associated microbes and infections	Possible mechanisms	Other associations
Ulcer disease, oesophagitis, gastritis, duodenitis, cholecystitis	*Helicobacter pylori* Upper gut fermenters (yeasts, aerobes, anaerobes – that is, abnormal gut microbiome)		
Pancreatitis	**Virus**: mumps, coxsackie, hepatitis B, cytomegalovirus, *Varicella zoster*, *Herpes simplex* **Bacteria**: *Mycoplasma*, *Legionella*, *Leptospira*, *Salmonella* **Fungi**: *Aspergillus* **Parasites**: *Toxoplasma*, *Cryptosporidium*, *Ascaris*	The pancreas is particularly susceptible because it has an open door (the bile duct) to the gut through which microbes from a fermenting gut can easily pass	Alcoholism Gall stones Also associated with selenium deficiency and poor antioxidant status
Hepatitis	Hepatitis B and C *Mycoplasma* *Yersinia*		
Crohn's disease	*Mycobacterium paratuberculosis avium* (MAP) – similar to Johne's disease in cattle	Acquired from milk – may be cured with antibiotics. Unfriendly gut microbes drive an inflammatory reaction	Also responds well to the PK diet Some cases are cured by antibiotics
Ulcerative colitis	Abnormal gut flora	Unfriendly gut microbes drive an inflammatory reaction	Responds well to the PK diet. Can be cured by faecal bacterio-therapy (see page 232)

Autoimmunity in general	Autoimmunity is directly associated with abnormal gut microbiome *Mycoplasma* is associated with many autoimmune conditions	Microbes spill over into the bloodstream, so antibodies are made against them; these cross-react with the self. This is called molecular mimicry. I think of this as allergy to microbes Gluten increases gut permeability and the risk of the above.	Sugar and refined carbohydrates Antibiotics Vaccination is a major risk factor for many autoimmune conditions, including type 1 diabetes Vitamin D deficiency also increases the risk The PK diet is an essential part of management
Autoimmunity specifics: multiple sclerosis (MS), thyroiditis, cardiomyopathy, primary biliary cirrhosis, rheumatoid arthritis, systemic lupus, Sjogren's syndrome	Epstein Barr virus is associated with at least 33 different autoimmune conditions All herpes viruses target the brain and immune system	Ditto	Ditto
Autoimmunity specifics: idiopathic thrombocytopenic purpura, systemic sclerosis, Crohn's disease, Guillain–Barré syndrome	*Helicobacter pylori*	Ditto	Ditto
Autoimmunity specifics: glomerular nephritis, rheumatic heart disease	Streptococcal infection (which can be treated by long-term, low-dose penicillin)	Ditto	Ditto
Autoimmunity specifics: narcolepsy, Guillain–Barré syndrome	Swine flu vaccination	Vaccination bypasses normal immune defences in the gut	

Disease	Associated microbes and infections	Possible mechanisms	Other associations
Brain conditions – all neurological disease may be associated with infection, including Alzheimer's, motor neurone disease, Parkinson's, CJD, multisystem atrophy	Many are related to abnormal gut microbiome, including autism, epilepsy, psychosis, schizophrenia, dementia, depression; *also* to *Borrelia, Mycoplasma, Ehrlichia, Anaplasma*	Nishihara[6] has shown where there is fermenting gut we have fermenting brain where neurotransmitters may be fermented into morphine, amphetamine and cocaine-like molecules. No wonder psychosis is a symptom – I would be psychotic with cocaine and crystal meth on the menu!	Responds well to the PK diet. Indeed, the starting point for treating all neurological and psychiatric disease is a PK diet. However, I would want to do extensive testing for 'stealth' microbes (see page 106) because conventional treatment for neurological degeneration is so limited
Kidney disease, interstitial cystitis and prostatitis	Abnormal gut flora *Bartonella*	This is not acute infection but an inflammatory process driven by microbes at levels lower than that which defines infection	Responds well to the PK diet and vitamin C to bowel tolerance. Some cases respond well to antibiotics
Respiratory problems – chronic sinusitis, rhinitis, pharyngitis, bronchitis, pneumonia etc	Infection (often *Mycoplasma*) and/or allergy to gut microbes	May present with halitosis	Pollution further drives inflammation. It is the total load – the total immune insult – which triggers inflammation
Eye disease – retinitis, optic neuritis, conjunctivitis, etc	*Chlamydia Bartonella Yersinia*		
Ear problems – otitis media, labyrinthitis	Streptococci and *Haemophilus* Flu and cold viruses		Often follow coughs, colds and influenza (see Chapter 18 for treatment)

At the moment, things do not look good.

See how numerous are my enemies and how fiercely they hate me!
Psalm 25:19, *The Bible* (New International Version)

Bur fear not… read on for the answers.

Chapter 3

The immune system is our standing army

Let us *'Begin at the beginning... and go on 'till... we... come to the end: then stop.'*
Alice in Wonderland, Lewis Carroll (27 January 1832 – 14 January 1898)

Beginning with an understanding of our natural defences and how the immune system works helps us to understand the principles of treatment. I think of the immune system as an army and that helps me when the immunologists descend into complex details which, I suspect, are iterated to show how clever they are! One does not have to be clever to get a grasp of the basic workings, which are as follows:

Table 3.1: Our natural defences and how they work

Defence	Mechanisms	Plus	Comments	Treatment implications
Physical barriers of defence against microbes	(1) Skin (2) Mucous membranes which line the airways, gut and perineum		The gut lining is less than perfect – microbes cross it easily and get into the bloodstream. We need friendly microbes in the gut to prevent serious disease	The skin needs fat to repel invaders; dry skin cracks and makes it easier for microbes to enter Carbohydrates feed unfriendly microbes Fibre feeds friendly microbes Fat feeds the immune system Probiotics displace unfriendly microbes

Secretions wash out microbes, assisted by coughing and sneezing	Saliva, tears, urine, sticky mucus in the mouth, gut, respiratory track and vagina...	...fortified by defensins, acid, bile, enzymes and fatty acids		The paleo-ketogenic (PK) diet results in healthy secretions Do not suppress symptoms and inhibit this natural expulsion of foreigners
White blood cells born in the bone marrow from 'mother' stem cells: neutrophils	The foot soldiers of our immune system – the 'Poor Bloody Infantry' of the *Wipers Times*, a trench magazine that was published by British soldiers fighting in the Ypres Salient during the First World War	Neutrophils take care of the invaders we have been dealing with for millions of years	Neutrophils do not learn new tricks and have no 'memory' of past experience; they do day-to-day sentry duty, firing off at sight or smell of invaders. These cells are born xenophobes!	All white cells need the correct raw materials to make them and the energy to allow them to fight A fever of one degree above your normal temperature is a symptom of energy generation being increased by 15% Keep warm, rest and save your energy to fight the good fight
		Neutrophils are also responsible for sweeping up the mess following an inflammatory war		This constitutes healing, which also requires sleep, energy and raw materials; convalescence is a serious matter
White blood cells: lymphocytes	Officer class B and T lymphocytes have to be educated. They can fight but can also tell the foot soldiers what to do	These are intelligent and necessary to deal with new, recently evolved invaders. They can be trained to do many different jobs and learn from others. These cells learn to become xenophobes!	They are supposed to learn good habits, such as fighting newly evolved microbes, *but* they may pick up *bad* habits, such as allergy or autoimmunity	Vaccination is supposed to train these officers correctly, but it may train them incorrectly and so switch on allergy, autoimmunity and neurodegeneration. We are seeing epidemics of all three in part due to our aggressive vaccination regimes

Defence	Mechanisms	Plus	Comments	Treatment implications
		With a new enemy, they take a little time to get started because they are learning	Having learned from experience they divide and their offspring also remember, so no time is wasted if the same enemy appears again	We call this immunity, but if they learn the wrong thing this may result in allergy and autoimmunity. Vaccination may provide temporary immunity, but a real infection confers life-long immunity
Killer T lymphocytes	Snipers	Specialise in killing cells that have been damaged by an invader by using CD8 to recognise such		Do not risk switching them on. Once switched on they are difficult to switch off. We do not have safe, targeted and reliably effective treatments for switching them off
Natural killer (NK) cells	Snipers	Specialise in killing cells occupied by virus	Also kill cancer cells	Ditto above – do not risk switching them on. Vitamin C and iodine kill with minimal activation of killer cells
Helper T cells	These help killer cells make good decisions about who to kill and who not to kill. They are like modern-day warfare 'target assessment officers'	This is so important – too much inflammation is as dangerous as too little	Too much inflammation is civil war – i.e. allergy and autoimmunity	Ditto
T regs (or T suppressor cells)	These regulate the immune response	They stop the soldiers from over-reacting…	…and guard against civil war	Ditto

B cells	Also help killer cells make good decisions by making antibodies	Ditto	Ditto	Ditto
Antibodies	These recognise the enemy, kill it directly and also…	…alert the immune system to switch on inflammation. They are 'look-outs'		
Prostaglandins Interferons Leucotrienes Eicosanoids Cytokines Chemokines	These allow foot soldiers and officers to communicate and send messages for help so are the 'messenger boys' or 'radio operators'…	… and develop the war zone that we call inflammation	Local inflammation means heat, redness, swelling, pain and loss of function. This is highly damaging to microbes but also to the self General inflammation will cause fever and severe fatigue	Inflammation must be followed by healing and repair. It also needs energy, raw materials and time. The PK diet is essential as are rest and sleep. Time is the great healer. We call this convalescence
Inflammation	This results when the immune system is activated	This is ideal for fighting invaders, but normal tissue gets caught up in friendly fire – this may be destructive	Too much general inflammation may result in a cytokine storm – this can kill you!	Many natural, nutritional, herbal and fungal products regulate this immune response
Complement	Bullets	Enhances all the above	Bullets can cause damage from friendly fire	
Vitamin C and iodine	Ideal ammunition …	… kill all bacteria, yeasts and viruses…	…and mop up their own damage	An essential treatment in all cases of infection

Defence	Mechanisms	Plus	Comments	Treatment implications
Antibiotics	Bullets which target bacteria	Plants and fungi which have survived billions of years of microbial attack are also rich in ammunition	Potential to damage the gut microbiome, but this is largely preventable with a PK diet, vitamin C and probiotics (see Chapters 6, 8, 9 and 37)	Their effects are greatly enhanced by attention to all the above
Antivirals	Bullets which target viruses	Ditto	Probably minimally damaging to the gut microbiome	Ditto
Antifungals	Bullets which target yeast	Ditto	Ditto	Ditto

Linguistic note: 'xenophobe' derives from the Ancient Greek words ξένος (*xenos*), meaning 'stranger' or 'foreigner, and φόβος (*phobos*), meaning 'fear'. Inside our bodies, xenophobia is a good thing, unless it turns on ourselves (autoimmunity). Outside our bodies, 'xenophobia' is a really good word for *Scrabble*!

There are many gaps in Table 3.1. This is because we do not know all the answers, neither do we understand the finely controlled checks and balances which keep our immune system in good shape. What we do know is that modern life is causing immune havoc – we have more chronic, degenerative disease, allergy, autoimmunity and cancer than ever before; the incidence of all these is rising fast. The risk of pandemic plague is high. The situation is far too complex for 'one drug' or 'one vaccination' measures. Do not wait for science to come up with a solution – it cannot and will not. Put in place the interventions now so that you are in pole position before hostilities begin.

Evolution has all the answers. We need to revert to an evolutionarily correct lifestyle or we will lose the arms race, but in addition to 'knowing ourselves' (understanding our immune systems) we must 'know the enemy', as Sun Tzu says in the *The Art of War*.

> *If you know the enemy and know yourself, you need not fear the result of a hundred battles. If you know yourself but not the enemy, for every victory gained you will also suffer a defeat. If you know neither the enemy nor yourself, you will succumb in every battle.*
>
> Sun Tzu, Chinese general (died 496 BC)

Our immune system has to be intelligent because the microbes attacking us are clever. Let's see how in the next chapter.

Chapter 4

Your enemy is fiendishly clever
An example of how cunning 'flu viruses are

Private Baldrick: I have a plan, sir.

Captain Blackadder: Really, Baldrick? A cunning and subtle one?

Private Baldrick: Yes, sir.

Captain Blackadder: As cunning as a fox who's just been appointed Professor of Cunning at Oxford University?

Blackadder Goes Forth,
'Goodbyeee'

Viruses are the Professors of Cunning, not the Baldricks!

These are the cunning steps that cold viruses (rhino viruses) and influenza viruses take to get into the body and how we can evade them. (Readers who are interested in the detailed mechanisms of herbs in respect of inhibition etc should consult the texts by Braun & Cohen and by Steven Buhner listed in the references.[7, 8, 9] It is beyond the scope of this book to give detailed explanations for all the various mechanisms of action, but, by way of example, references are included below with respect to Chinese skullcap.)

Table 4.1: Cunning steps viruses take and ways to thwart them

The cunning steps that rhino viruses and influenza viruses take to get into the body...	...and what we can do to slow or prevent this happening
When we inhale, we can acquire the influenza virus – it lands on the mucous membranes which line our respiratory tract	Some is coughed up and swallowed. We need an acid bath in our stomach to kill this. Increase your vitamin C to 10 grams every hour
	Kill the virus directly before it enters the body with an iodine salt pipe (see First aid box – Appendix 1, page 215), zinc, selenium and/or *Echinacea angustifolia*
Just like a ship coming into port, the virus docks onto a receptor on the membranes of our cells called haemagglutinin. This allows the 'terrorist' virus to lock on and thereafter to start the process of entering the body	Chinese skullcap mushroom (*Scutellaria baicalensis*) inhibits this process. For inhibition of neuroaminidase inhibitors the exact mechanism is complex but interested readers can read the superb article by Hour et al (2013)[10]; for its action as an inhibitor of cytokines see the articles on Examine.com[11]
Having stuck to the dockside, the virus releases an enzyme, neuraminidase, which softens the dock wall so that the lock gates open. For our terrorist virus these really are the gates to heaven!	Neuraminidase inhibitors slow this process – e.g. herbals such as Chinese skullcap, elderberry, liquorice, rhodiola, ginger and isatis
	Also prescription drugs such as Tamiflu and Relenza work this way
Once inside the cell the virus wants its own bed and control centre. As the gates of heaven open, such a bed and control centre – called a 'vacuole' – are created	

The cunning steps that rhino viruses and influenza viruses take to get into the body…	…and what we can do to slow or prevent this happening
The virus sticks to the lining of the vacuole and creates a tiny pore through which it can direct further affairs to its own advantage. This pore is called an M2 ion channel	*Lomatium* is a herb which has the common names of biscuitroot, Indian parsley and desert parsley. It is a powerful inhibitor of M2 development. The M2 ion channel is specific to influenza A which is the most dangerous form of 'flu The drug amantadine is meant to work by inhibiting this, but resistance is common since this drug has been so widely used in the poultry industry that it has been rendered pretty useless for humans. In the case of influenza B, the BM2 protein has ion channel activity,[12] which is not inhibited by *Lomatium*. More than 200 different viruses are known to cause the symptoms of the common cold, but an estimated 30-35% of adult colds are caused by rhinoviruses – see Atkinson et al (2016) for a comprehensive review.[13]
Once the M2 pore is open, the virus uses this porthole to hijack the cell machinery and direct it to make more virus. (Whoever said viruses were not intelligent?) The cell is sucked dry by these vicious demands, becomes exhausted and dies and the new young terrorists move into the next cell	Vitamin C takes up the protein coats being manufactured by the virus nucleic acid, thus preventing the assembly of new viral units. Cells expand, rupture and die, but there are no virus particles available to enter and infect new cells. Once the virus has invaded a cell, vitamin C contributes to its breakdown through the enzyme adenosine deaminase, which converts adenosine to inosine. Purines are formed which are catabolised (broken down) and cannot be used to make more viral nucleic acid.
As lung cells die, the lungs do not work so well and all the symptoms of lung disease and infection strike – malaise, sore throat, cough, mucus, shortness of breath and eventually pneumonia…	

Throughout all the above, the virus additionally manipulates the body's immune system to its own advantage in two ways. The longer the virus can hold off effective resistance the more it can replicate – in particular it: 1. prevents type 1 interferon production using NS1 protein	Liquorice upregulates type 1 interferon production
2. inhibits the white cell response	Increase white cell responses with zinc, iodine, selenium, vitamin C, liquorice and elderberry
With too much of the above (i.e. prevention of type 1 interferon production and inhibition of the white cell response), the immune system flips into a 'cytokine storm'. It's as if the body realises it's been duped and sends in the atomic bomb. But this can be counterproductive and the 'friendly fire' can overwhelm and cause terrible tissue damage	This was a major cause of death during the 1918 Spanish 'flu epidemic which killed an estimated 52 million worldwide – about 3% of the world's population.[14]
Indeed, the influenza virus also moves into and hijacks immune cells, causing them to pour out cytokines and chemokines. Again, some of this action is inappropriate	Inhibit overly toxic cytokines, such as TNF alpha, with Chinese skullcap, elderberry, liquorice and *Cordyceps*. It is wonderful how these herbs multitask. This partly explains why resistance to herbs does not arise – because the chances of any microbe simultaneously acquiring resistant genes to multiple factors is vanishingly small, especially when they (the herbs) are not used in the poultry production industry!
	Mice that cannot produce TNF alpha, a cytokine, have fewer symptoms and lower mortality when infected with the Spanish 'flu virus
Another cytokine – TGF beta2 – may be overproduced	Inhibit this cytokine with *Astragalus*, Chinese skullcap and Japanese honeysuckle
Another cytokine – HMGB1 – may be overproduced (Don't worry about the names – I don't because I can never remember them and remembering them does not change what needs to be done)	Inhibit this cytokine with *Angelica sinensis*, liquorice, green tea and quercetin. In severe cases, prescription antivirals, steroids, NSAIDs and antibiotics (except, oddly, minocycline) have no effect, but herbs do Oxygen can be vital to allow patients to survive

The cunning steps that rhino viruses and influenza viruses take to get into the body...	...and what we can do to slow or prevent this happening
There are inevitably dead cells (killed by virus) and collateral damage from friendly fire. Drainage lymph nodes in the lungs enlarge to clear up the mess. A test for cell-free DNA taken at this stage would show a high result because so many cell walls have been ruptured	Good quality sleep greatly improves the brain's ability to heal and repair itself as the glymphatic system is activated in non-REM sleep. Improve lymphatic drainage with red root, immortal and pleurisy root
Viruses like sugar too – the saying 'feed a cold, starve a fever' should be 'starve a cold, starve a fever'. The body has more than enough fat reserves to power itself for a few days	Eat a PK diet. All infections are encouraged by sugar and carbs. Do not eat that bunch of grapes, however lovingly they have been purchased. Intravenous glucose during 'flu substantially increases viral load and worsens symptoms. I suspect sugar feeds the cytokine storm as it is so pro-inflammatory

Viruses are no joke – just look at the derivation of the word: from the Latin 'virus', meaning a venomous substance, poison or slimy liquid. The Latin is probably earlier derived from the proto-Indian European – 'weis' – to melt away, to flow, used in the context of foul fluids and poisons. But here is a joke anyway:

A virus walks into a bar. The bartender says, 'We don't serve viruses here.' The virus says, 'Well, you're not a very good host.'
Later that day, having been rejected once, the virus returns...
It walks into the bar again. The bartender says, 'We don't serve viruses here.'
The virus replaces the bartender and says, 'Now we do.'

In the next chapter, let's look at the signs that tell us that our enemy is among us and that we are losing the arms race.

Chapter 5

We are already losing the arms race

The fight against infection is not a battle; it is a war. Unlike King Pyrrhus of Epirus, who won the battle of Heraclea in 280 BC by beating the Romans but lost the war (hence a 'Pyrrhic victory'), we must concentrate on winning the war. And this war is equivalent to trench warfare (long and slow), not a Blitzkrieg (literally, like lightning).

The war is waged throughout life and is also like siege warfare, with us humans defending our castle and the microbes fighting to get in. Babies are already losing this battle. Caesarian sections and bottle-feeding mean they are not correctly inoculated or fed. Oral thrush, a fungal infection of the mouth, is commonplace. Doctors appear completely unconcerned, but already the first battle has been lost. Fermenting mouths lead to fermenting guts. The gut is leaky – microbes in the gut then get into the body (this is called 'bacterial translocation' – see page 31) and we now know these are driving a wide range of pathologies.[15]

Gobs and guts

The vast majority of microbes get into our bodies through inhalation or ingestion (with food or drink). Those inhaled adhere to the sticky mucus that lines the respiratory tract, are coughed up and swallowed. All such microbes should end up in the acid bath of the stomach which should kill them. Maintaining an acid stomach is an essential defence. Western diets and lifestyles upset this natural and highly desirable defence mechanism in many ways:

1. **High carbohydrate diets** result in foods being fermented instead of digested. The microbes which do this cause a low-grade inflammation of the stomach lining which results in leaky gut. As fast as the cells lining the stomach wall pump acid into the lumen (interior of the stomach), the acid leaks back out.

2. **Allergy** – the common allergens are dairy products and gluten grains; the resulting low-grade inflammation creates the same problem as above.

3. **Gluten** – We know gluten damages the tight junctions between cells and renders the gut leaky. This fact alone make gluten unsafe for anyone to eat. I consider it to be a poison.

4. **Snacking** – The stomach has a chance, when empty between meals, to restore normal acidity. Constant snacking or consumption of sweet foods and drinks feeds microbes directly and prevents the stomach cleaning itself.

Certain drugs can also be an issue as is discussed in Chapter 12.

An acid stomach is an essential part of digesting proteins and absorbing micronutrients such as iron and vitamin B12. All of these proteins and micronutrients are essential for good quality skin, good quality mucus and a good immune system. Our standing army is weakened by lack of raw materials.

Mucus may be snot to you, but it's my bread and butter.
> Dr David Freed, Reader in Immunology MB ChB MD CBiol MIBiol

---

Editorial note – I happened to be drinking a nice cup of green tea at the very time I read this wonderful quote – I nearly choked there and then! Craig

---

There is much more detail of the above mechanisms in our books *Sustainable Medicine – whistleblowing on 21st century medical practice* and *Prevent and Cure Diabetes – delicious diets not dangerous drugs*, also published by Hammersmith Books.

Genitals and gnats

Sexually transmitted disease and biting insects represent two further major routes of infection whereby microbes can dodge our first lines of defence (see Chapter 14, Use your brain).

How do you know when you are losing the arms race?

Know your enemy...and learn about his favourite sport.
Nelson Mandela (18 July 1918 – 5 December 2013)

Here the 'sport' is how the enemy plays the game – knowing about this means that we can work out ways to beat him at his own game. More of this follows in Chapters 18 onwards, and also see Chapters 2 and 4. In the meantime, symptoms are, as ever, our clues, and there are several common symptoms which indicate that you are losing the arms race, and which are now so commonplace that they are generally accepted as normal:

1. **Dental plaque** – This is the tough shield that bacteria throw up in order to make themselves at home on our teeth (an example of 'biofilm'). It cannot even be scrubbed off with a tooth brush; the dentist has to get out his chisel.

> I once gave my dentist a black eye whilst under gas for an extraction. Luckily, he found the whole thing very amusing – being taken down by a 7-year-old boy! Craig

   High-carbohydrate diets feed bacteria in the mouth directly, but sugar in the bloodstream will also spill over into saliva. This is why plaque first appears on the inner surface of the lower incisor teeth, right opposite the salivary duct. If you are not sure if you have plaque, use disclosing fluid which stains plaque pink.

2. **'BO' (body odour)** – Normal sweat is odourless. However, high-carbohydrate diets result in high blood sugar; this sugar spills over into sweat on the skin, where it is fermented by skin microbes. These ferments are foul smelling. I think of this as farting skin!

> The word 'fart' is one of the oldest in the English lexicon.

Interestingly this leads to an interesting cure for BO: the skin is sterilised with topical antimicrobials then inoculated with donor microbes from the armpit of a non-smeller, ideally a family member.

> According to *The Alphabet of Manliness* (by Maddox), the assigning of blame for farting is part of a ritual of behaviour. This may involve deception and a back and forth rhyming game – for example, 'He who smelt it, dealt it' and 'He who denied it, supplied it'. Having a dog to blame helps too!

3. **Yeast infections:** dandruff, fungal nails, a tendency to athlete's foot, perineal thrush or ringworm – yeast loves sugar.

4. **A tendency to coughs and colds** – These have become accepted and inevitable parts of Western life. However, to get such is symptomatic of failed defences and failed immunity. You will know when you have put enough in place to win this arms race because coughs and colds will become a thing of the past. In this respect, vitamin C is a major player.

5. **Being apple shaped** – Fat is laid down where the immune system is busy. Fat laid round the gut means energy is required for the immune system to fight back against microbes in the fermenting gut.

> **Note:** Research done by Professor Caroline Pond at Oxford University has shown that the immune system is fat-loving. Wild animals, if they have a food glut, will first deposit fat around lymph nodes where energy is needed for immune activity. So, fat deposited around the gut (apple-shaped) indicates inflammation there.[16]

6. **Joint and muscle aches and stiffness** – There is a general assumption that microbes in the gut are contained there. Wrong! Gut microbes are miniscule compared with human cells and they all too easily spill over into the bloodstream. This is called bacterial translocation, as mentioned above. If these microbes are evolutionarily correct, so our innate immune system has been seeing and dealing with them for years, then there is no problem. However, new microbes, which may come from inoculation by vaccination or the upper fermenting gut, may not be recognised as friendly. Remember, white cells are xenophobes; they are born and educated to attack foreigners! New-to-the-immune-system microbes may get stuck in departments where there has been tissue damage and scarring. We all damage ourselves during life, with scar tissue in our joints, tendons, connective tissue and muscles. These new-to-the-immune-system microbes have the potential to switch on inflammation, and this is characterised by friction (stiffness) and pain. So often I see people with chronic pain triggered by injury for which painkillers for life are prescribed. A paleo-ketogenic (PK) diet, perhaps with natural or prescription antimicrobials, can cure the problem.

If you suffer from any one of the above, then you know you are already harbouring billions of unfriendly microbes which, with time and/or opportunity, will invade deeper into your tissues and drive one or several of the nasty pathologies detailed in Chapter 2. Recognise these symptoms as red warning flags – they all represent stages of disease which can probably be reversed. Do not try to suppress the symptoms because this further inhibits the immune system's war against infection. For example, it is no coincidence that drugs for arthritis substantially increase the risk of heart disease and dementia. As you can see, there is a clear, biologically plausible explanation for this – drugs for arthritis suppress the immune system and we have seen in Chapter 2 how infections drive heart disease and dementia; these infections will have an easier passage if the immune system is suppressed. Do not wait until you have received your diagnosis of cancer, heart disease or dementia before acting. Recognise that the writing is on the wall, that the ship is heading for the rocks or that you are heading for a fall. Preferably all three! See trouble wherever you look and act now.

A stitch in time saves nine.

Old English proverb

As Sun Tzu said in *The Art of War* (Chapter 3), we now know 'ourselves' (our immune system) and we also know the 'enemy' (and the signs that he is winning), and so now we must begin to learn the tactics of this war – tactics that will enable us to achieve victory.

Part II

The starting point is
to improve our defences

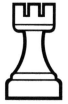

Chapter 6

The general approach to avoiding and treating infection

I: Improve the defences – Diet, micronutrients and sleep

Let food and micronutrients be thy medicine and medicine be thy food and micronutrients.

With apologies to Hippocrates, 'Father of Modern Medicine' (460 – 370 BC)

Editor's comment: I am following a rich tradition of misquoting or misattributing quotations to bend them for my own purposes. A favourite, often attributed to Marilyn Monroe, but actually by Laurel Thatcher Ulrich, a professor from Harvard University is:

'*…well-behaved women seldom make history…*'.

Sarah is trying her best here, thankfully: Craig.

(That is the first time anyone has called me well-behaved. I told you he was a gentleman: Sarah)

Microbes (with a few very rare exceptions) can only survive if fed with carbohydrates. By contrast, animal cells can run on fats. Animal cells can also run on carbohydrates and this dual-fuel ability brings huge evolutionary benefits. Traditionally, humans have switched to carbohydrate burning during the autumn to allow them to benefit from the carbohydrate bonanza of this natural harvest-time, which allows the laying down of fat. This brought the essential survival values of insulation against cold winter weather and a pantry against lean times. Winter, spring and early summer diets were fat- and fibre-based – in other words, ketogenic. Westerners with modern food supplies live in a permanent autumn. We love this because carbohydrates are so addictive, but eating like this is also so dangerous as we explain in much more detail in our books *Prevent and Cure Diabetes – delicious diets not dangerous drugs* and *The PK Cookbook*.

I believe this ability to run on fats was an early tool that allowed animals to get sufficiently far ahead in the arms race to evolve. Regardless of whether this is correct, the fact remains that diets based on fat and fibre are unfriendly to invading microbes. This is in direct contrast to diets based on sugar and starch. These foods actively feed and encourage microbes. Diabetics are particularly susceptible to infection because of their high levels of blood sugar. Babies get oral thrush because this yeast (candida) happily ferments sugar in milk – even breast milk will be high in sugar if Mum is eating a Western diet. Artificial Western bottle-feed is even sweeter.

Indeed, I suspect it is high-carb diets that, if not creating the problem, are surely contributing to antibiotic resistance. This is the greatest problem in hospitals partly because patients are fed high-carb diets – cheap, convenient, soft and addictive – which feed microbes and encourage their survival. It is intellectually risible to feed the very microbes you are trying to kill. A dose of antibiotic kills a percentage of the target bacteria, but a carb meal between doses helps microbes to recover. Given sugar, bacteria and yeast can double their numbers every 20 minutes. It is an irony that every hospital bed has a bowl of fruit adjacent to it when fruit sugar is as pernicious as the white stuff.

The starting point for preventing and treating all infection is the paleo-ketogenic (PK) diet. This aims to replicate evolutionarily correct diets so we can live to our full potential in terms of quality and quantity of life. The principles of this diet are:

- Fuel yourself with fat and fibre, not sugar and starch. Nourish yourself and starve the microbes.
- Eat two good meals a day – no snacking.
- Avoid dairy products which, contrary to perceived wisdom, are not natural foods. When challenged on this, I point out that opium is a natural plant but not one generally perceived as a health food. Dairy products are common allergens and are also growth promoters.
- Avoid gluten grains. Gluten is a toxic protein and a common allergen (like dairy products) and creates a leaky gut. Allergy is estimated to afflict at least 30% of Westerners. The protein content of modern wheat may be 80% gluten compared with primitive wheat, where it was 20%.

- Be sure your diet is rich in micronutrients. Our book *The PK Cookbook* gives details of the additional micronutrients we require to compensate for the deficiencies induced by Western agriculture. An essential part of this is 'Sunshine salt' – a salt which contains all the essential minerals, plus a good dose of vitamin D and vitamin B_{12}, and helps correct the deficiencies of Western foods. Combine this with a good daily multivitamin and you will have all the major micronutrients in your diet.
- Be sure your diet is rich in spices and herbs. All plants and fungi have survived millions of years of evolution using their own particular form of chemical warfare. They too fight an arms race against microbes. All plants and fungi contain natural antiviral, antibacterial, antifungal, antiparasitic and anti-worm toxins. Happily, many taste wonderful – again, that is no surprise as the brain has learned to seek out foods that are good for our survival and it encourages us to eat them by giving us a hugely pleasurable experience. I do not think it matters much which herbs and spices you eat so long as you eat a lot of them.
- Be sure your diet is low in addictive potential. Western lifestyles are dangerously addictive – you can see many laid out when you stop to refuel your car – chocolate, sweets, crisps, cigarettes, caffeine, alcohol, gambling and sex magazines to name a few. As any addict will tell you, one addiction tends to switch on another. I believe that sugar is more addictive than, and more dangerous than, smoking.
- Be sure your diet is high in fibre. Fibre is fermented by friendly, evolutionarily correct microbes in the lower gut (large bowel) into many helpful products. These include heat, short-chain fatty acids (another fat fuel supply) and essential vitamins, such as vitamin K. Friendly microbes train the immune system to respond appropriately and displace unfriendly microbes from the gut. These actions are all highly protective against infection.

All the above:
- inhibit the upper fermenting gut[17] – this further improves digestion and absorption of food and prevents leaky gut; and
- reduce the toxic load of Western diets in the gut, a load which has the potential to overload the liver.

There is much more detail about the *why* of this diet in our book *Prevent and Cure Diabetes – delicious diets not dangerous drugs* and, perhaps more importantly, *The PK Cookbook* gives you the *how*. This may be a difficult diet to initiate and you may need the intellectual imperatives and practical details of the above two books to get started. It may be no consolation to you to hear that I had to work for 35 years in general medical practice, treat an estimated 20,000 patients and, with the wonderful Craig, write four books in order to establish the diet for myself. Having arrived, I now feel genuinely sorry for people who are not doing this diet and thereby consigning themselves to a shortened lifetime with miserable potential. I do now understand the full potential of addiction, which does not just result in poor eating habits but defends them with humour and wit!

One of the problems of waking up in the morning without a hangover is that you know it's the best you are going to feel for the rest of the day.

Reputedly overheard at a dinner party conversation circa 1973,
Leonard Parkin ITV News presenter (1929 – 1993)

We put together *The PK Cookbook* so that, like Craig and me, you can enjoy a rich and varied diet with gorgeous bread and dairy alternatives. To give you an idea of this, here is a typical daily PK diet:

Breakfast – choose from/mix and match:
 Coconut yoghurt (e.g. Coyo)
 PK porridge or muesli (based on linseed and coconut – see *PK Cookbook*)
 PK toast (this is based on linseed, but looks and slices like a small brown loaf –
  see *PK Cookbook*) with vegan 'butter', e.g. coconut spread
 Boiled eggs
 Fresh, frozen, cured or tinned fish and shell fish
 Fresh, frozen, cured or tinned meat: salami, pate
 Vegan cheese
 Omelette with mushrooms
 Fry up – bacon, eggs, PK bread fried in lard, sausage (high-fat, rusk-free), liver,
  black pudding – see *The PK Cookbook*
 Last night's PK vegetables (low-carb) fried in lard, coconut butter or palm oil – see
  PK Cookbook

No snacks: Quench thirst with water. Use coffee and tea judiciously.

Lunch

None – have a kip instead.

Editor's note – It's called 'power napping': Craig

Supper

Starters:

Olives, PK nuts – e.g. Brazils, pecans (some nuts are high in carbohydrate, including my favourites, cashews and pistachio nuts, so beware! Relative levels are listed in *The PK Cookbook*)

Large bowl of sauerkraut

PK toast with above breakfast suggestions

Large bowl of salad with mayonnaise or French dressing

Main course:

Meat, poultry, fish cooked with lots of herbs and spices

Abundant green vegetables

Puddings:

Berries with coconut milk

PK ice cream (see *The PK Cookbook*)

Dark 80%+ chocolate

As I constantly reiterate, to the boredom of my friends and the irritation of my daughters, there is little point in progressing to other interventions until the PK diet is established. There are further powerful interventions we can make to improve our defences, help the immune system and kill the enemy, but the power of these interventions is hugely compromised if we are feeding our foes at the same time. Killing and feeding microbes simultaneously provides the perfect breeding and training grounds for tough microbes. Combine this with our deteriorating immune function and we create the perfect storm. When this perfect storm will come and what form it will take (bird 'flu, swine 'flu, SARS, MARS, Ebola virus, Lassa fever, Rift Valley fever to name a few) is not known. What we do know for certain is that come it will and we do not currently have the necessary defences to prevent deaths. Those people with good defences will have a much better chance of survival. I want me, my family, my friends and patients to survive…and enjoy life to the maximum potential.

It really is a case of the 'survival of the fittest', which, by the way, is another often-misattributed quotation. Herbert Spencer first used this phrase, after reading Charles Darwin's *On the Origin of Species*. Spencer drew parallels between his economic theories and Darwin's biological ones, saying:

This survival of the fittest, which I have here sought to express in mechanical terms, is that which Mr Darwin has called 'natural selection', or the preservation of favoured races in the struggle for life.

Alfred Russel Wallace suggested to Darwin using Spencer's new phrase of the 'survival of the fittest' as an alternative to 'natural selection', and Darwin adopted the phrase in *The Variation of Animals and Plants under Domestication* published in 1868. Herbert Spencer – English philosopher, biologist, anthropologist and sociologist (27 April 1820 – 8 December 1903) Charles Darwin – English naturalist and geologist (12 February 1809 – 19 April 1882), Alfred Russel Wallace – Welsh naturalist, explorer, geographer, anthropologist and biologist (8 January 1823 – 7 November 1913)

Sleep

It is during sleep that we heal and repair. Most of the deaths from friendly fire in the Gulf War came from sleep-deprived soldiers making bad decisions. Our immune white-cell soldiers are the same – they too need sleep. Any animal deprived of sleep for long enough will die. I was intrigued to learn that the cause of death in such cases is septicaemia from microbes invading from the gut. It is also my experience, and that of others, that there is a recognisable death smell that emanates from someone slowly gasping their last. I suspect this reflects this same early septicaemia.

We need both REM (rapid eye movement) sleep and non-REM sleep. It is during the latter where at least two important functions are performed. Firstly, we sort out the experiences of the day and memorise those that afford survival benefit. Secondly, the glymphatics (a functional waste clearance pathway in the brain and spinal cord) dust and clean the brain, eliminating toxins such as the waste products of metabolism. This dusting and cleaning may include the amyloid of prion protein – the infectious particle that is associated with Alzheimer's, Parkinson's, motor neurone disease, nvCJD ('mad cow' disease) and probably multi-system atrophy. There is now clear evidence that lack of non-REM sleep is a risk factor for, *and* cause of, Alzheimer's – this makes for a hideous vicious cycle. The interested reader should read the medical papers listed in the Reference section (page 222) concerning the issue of non-REM sleep and its importance.[18, 19, 20, 21, 22, 23]

But let's put it simply: if you do not get sufficient good quality sleep you will develop neurological disease.

It is during REM sleep that the brain solves problems. It does this by making all sorts of neurological cross-party chit chat. This manifests with dreams where the peculiar and bizarre are guaranteed. Fortunately during REM sleep our muscles are paralysed so we cannot act out our dreams. In non-REM sleep, the muscles are not paralysed and although rare, this can lead to catastrophe, for example in one case of a man who, whilst fast asleep, murdered his step-mother; I too have had similarly psychotic, delusional dreams but happily for my mother-in-law, Jean, paralysis prevailed. On the other hand, Craig, as a boy, was a prolific sleep-walker, who once emerged from his parents' kitchen with a plate of bacon and eggs, all cooked in his sleep – his parents had simply watched him and let him be…and then he went back upstairs…plate and frying pan unwashed!) From a practical standpoint, should you ever have a problem that is bothering you, sleep on it. I always do. On waking you will almost always find the problem is solved.

The sleep of Westerners is impaired in quantity and quality:

- **Quantity**: Many people do not allow themselves the necessary time for sleep. The average sleep requirement is eight to nine hours in bed between 9.30 pm and 6.30 am (more in winter, less in summer and, yes, the time of night is also critical. Do not think you can catch up at weekends – you simply do not get the quality of sleep required). However, the actual average sleep time for Westerners is seven and a half hours. This results in a ratchetting down of health, which is often ascribed to ageing.

- **Quality:** This is impaired by addiction, especially to sugar, alcohol and caffeine. This may be compounded when the addiction is used to suppress the hugely unpleasant symptoms of stress. Sleep should be undisturbed by adrenalin, mouth-breathing and snoring, light, noise, heat, infrasound and electromagnetic radiation (wifi, mobiles, computers, TVs and cordless phones – ban them all from the bedroom).

We now have our first weapons in this war: diet, micronutrients and sleep. Let us now learn more and increase our armoury!

Chapter 7

The general approach to avoiding and treating infection
II. Energy delivery mechanisms

We need a plentiful supply of energy to fight infection for at least two reasons.

Reason 1: To power our immune system

The immune system is our standing army. Armies are hugely demanding of energy. How do I know this? Give a normal person a dose of 'flu and they become bedbound. Every spare ATP molecule is thrown at our dashing officers and gallant foot soldiers to fight the good fight. As Richard Straub has noted, 'During acute infections, such as sepsis, the total energy expenditure of the immune system can increase by 30-60%.'[24]

Interestingly, this complete depletion of energy really does seem to happen more with men than women, and hence the famous label of 'man 'flu'. More on this later, but researchers at Royal Holloway, University of London, have recently investigated this gender difference. Francesco Ubeda comments that:

> *Viruses may be evolving to be less dangerous to women, looking to preserve the female population. The virus wants to be passed from mother to child, either through breastfeeding, or just through giving birth.*

Dr Ubeda's co-author, Professor Vincent Jansen, postulates that a virus might be able to tell if its host is a man or a woman by detecting hormonal and other differences, although it is not yet clear how exactly it would do this.[25] The researchers used a variation of the classic SIR model of infection transmission (an area of mathematical biology – please direct questions to Craig, as he studied this at university and/or consult the Reference list on page 223).[26, 27]

Editorial note: Given that this was a mathematical model looking at theoretical possibilities only, I am content to continue with the man 'flu jokes for the time being! – Craig – sigh

---

Reason 2: To keep warm

Wrap up warm, darling, or you will catch your death of cold

Mother was right…again! Keeping body temperature just right is an essential survival mechanism. Running too hot wastes energy and would have reduced primitive man's chances of surviving a winter or famine. However, running too cold is a risk factor for infection. The body needs to hold its core temperature at exactly 37 degrees centigrade, with fluctuations of no more than 0.3 of a degree.

In the paper 'Temperature-dependent innate defense against the common cold virus limits viral replication at warm temperature in mouse airway cells',[28] researchers showed that temperature alters the ability of the airway cells to mount an effective innate immune response against rhinovirus, the microbe responsible for the common cold. Indeed, these Yale-based researchers concluded that a vital natural defence against infection is simply to keep warm.

There are other mechanisms at work here too. Indeed, the burning of brown fat in the newborn baby is an essential part of survival to keep him warm – this kills the microbes that inevitably invade through the fresh, juicy free lunch of an umbilical cord. Lambs born on the hill who get cold almost always die from liver abscesses as infection tracks in from the cord. (I know this because during my years of sheep farming I used to cut them open to see why they had succumbed. Thereafter, if I found a cold newborn lamb on the hill I would bring him into the kitchen to warm up – but without an injection of antibiotic it invariably died. My daughter Ruth commented that the lambs started life in the bottom oven and finished life in the top!)

Anyone who is run-down, stressed, starved, old and cold, over-worked and/or over-tired is at greater risk of infection. It is amazing how many people crash and burn at Christmas, or can date the onset of their post-viral fatigue from this period.

If energy delivery mechanisms are impaired, then the immune system is starved of energy and unable to fight effectively. Being cold is an invitation for microbes to invade. An analogy I constantly use is to liken energy delivery mechanisms to a car. If there are problems in any one of the areas listed in Table 7.1 then energy delivery is impaired. This results in immune suppression.

Table 7.1: Energy delivery

Car	Human	Notes
Fuel – the correct sort	Need fat and fibre, *not* sugar and carbs	See our books *Prevent and Cure Diabetes – delicious diets not dangerous drugs* and *The PK Cookbook* (PK = 'Paleo-ketogenic')
Engine	Mitochondria – these take fuel, burn it in the presence of oxygen to provide the energy molecule ATP	See our book *Diagnosis and Treatment of Chronic Fatigue Syndrome and Myalgic Encephalitis: it's mitochondria, not hypochondria*. Mitochondria may go slow because they lack the raw materials to work or because they are inhibited by toxins.
Fuel pump Air intake	Heart, lungs and blood supply	Deliver fuel and oxygen to the engine (mitochondria). It is pretty obvious that fatigue will result from heart failure, lung failure or anaemia
Accelerator pedal	Thyroid gland	Consultant endocrinologist Dr Kenneth Blanchard estimates at least 20% of Western women are hypothyroid. See www.naturalhealthworldwide.com – Natural Health Worldwide ('NHW') – for access to DIY blood tests. These are pinprick tests that can be done by patients on their own at home without the need for doctors or nurses to draw blood
Gear box	Adrenal gland	Allows one to gear up energy delivery according to demand. The output of stress hormones is greatly ramped up during infection. An adrenal stress test is a good test and available through NHW – again this can be done by patients on their own at home without the need for intervention by doctors or nurses – this is a saliva test

Car	Human	Notes
Servicing, healing and repair	Sleep	On average we need 8-9 hours of quality sleep in every 24. Most Westerners are chronically sleep deprived. Sleep-deprived rats die from gut microbes causing septicaemia. They do not have the energy to maintain their gut defences. We need to be as disciplined about sleep as diet – both are so important for 'rude good health'
Catalytic converter and exhaust pipe	Liver and kidneys	Liver failure and kidney failure also cause fatigue
Driver	Brain	So important and so difficult to get a good balance of physical, mental and emotional work and rest. See our book *Diagnosis and Treatment of Chronic Fatigue Syndrome and Myalgic Encephalitis: it's mitochondria, not hypochondria* for suggestions

The symptom of fatigue

We have the symptom of fatigue for very good reasons – it protects the body from itself. We are productive and have fun when we spend energy. Without fatigue we would work and have fun day and night, but within two weeks we would all be dead. After the First World War, a strain of 'flu (known as 'Spanish 'flu') swept through Europe and the wider world, killing in excess of 50 million people worldwide. Some people sustained neurological damage from this virus; in some it wiped out the sleep centre in their brain. This meant they were unable to sleep at all. All these poor people were dead within two weeks and this was the first solid scientific evidence that sleep is more essential for life than food and water.

Listen to your body, hear that it is tired and take the necessary difficult steps to correct this. If you live life constantly 'on the edge' then you will have no reserves to cope with the infectious stress. I liken this to walking along the white cliffs of Dover. Walk too near the edge and a puff of wind will send you on a damaging crash to the beach. If you survive, crawling back up the cliffs is difficult, time consuming and painful. Walk a few yards away from the edge and if you are blown over, you will land on the soft, green grass and it is no matter to stand up, dust yourself down and carry on.

Core temperature

The actual core temperature is a measure of total energy delivery mechanisms and this is a very useful clinical tool. Like a car we need the correct fuel in the tank (ketones), a good engine (mitochondria), the accelerator pedal (thyroid) and the gear box (adrenal) set just right. I think of this as conducting the CFS's orchestra – all four players need to be in place at the right time, volume and rhythm to get a melody that will power you for life.[29] The sum total output of energy is reflected by core temperature and this is a very useful guide for you, the conductor of your orchestra.

Indeed, there is a subtle and complex interplay between the adrenal and thyroid glands which control energy delivery mechanisms so they precisely match energy demands. Any inaccuracy and energy is wasted or not available for essential services. Thyroid hormones base load and set the average core temperature whilst adrenal hormones adjust energy delivery on a second by second (adrenalin) and minute by minute (cortisol) basis. Indeed, adrenalin and cortisol increase mitochondrial output by over 200% – that is why people often feel so well with an adrenalin buzz and/or whilst taking steroids – but then there is payback time later.

Put simply, if your body is constantly running cold you will be far more susceptible to infection.

Do not mask symptoms with addiction

The sensation of limitless energy is a delight. With endless energy one can conquer the world singlehandedly (well, I thought I could!). This is what drives the hope of youth. Declining energy delivery is paralleled by the realism of middle age. Addictions give us a temporary sensation of limitless energy and that is why we can never have enough of them.

Foods such as bread, cereals, biscuits, crisps, fruit, sweets, chocolate and dairy products are addictive. These foods provide a very short-term, addictive buzz of energy. And there is a particular vicious cycle here because these are the very foods which result in metabolic syndrome, fermenting gut, allergy and micronutrient deficiencies, all of which deplete energy. Worse still, the symptoms these foods create mean that people turn to other addictions to relieve those symptoms – to caffeine, nicotine and possibly others. (For much more on this, see our books *Diagnosis and Treatment of CFS/ME – it's mitochondria, not hypochondria* and *Prevent and Cure Diabetes – delicious diets not dangerous drugs*.)

In the short term, addiction masks the symptom of fatigue and this allows us to ignore essential you-are-running-out-of-energy symptoms to, perhaps, achieve great things. Addiction masks other unpleasant symptoms which are also a result of poor energy delivery mechanisms and which we collectively recognise as 'feeling stressed'.

In the medium term, addiction causes immune suppression and puts us at risk of acute infection.

In the long term, addiction greatly increases the risk of all diseases, from dementia and diabetes to cancer and coronaries. Indeed, as dear reader you will see throughout this book, chronic infection drives many of these conditions.

Do not succumb to the false energy of these addictions, but rather concentrate on the sustainable energy of the PK diet, a good micronutrient status, refreshing sleep and all the energy delivery mechanisms mentioned above. As noted before, this arms race is a marathon, not a sprint, and you will not last long using short-term hits.

As C S Lewis wrote, in a different context, but somehow it chimes with our key point here, these addictions are:

...the sweet poison of the false infinite...

Perelandra by CS Lewis (29 November 1898 – 22 November 1963)

© copyright CS Lewis Pte Ltd 1944.

Chapter 8

The gut microbiome:
inoculate the gut, feed it and train the immune system

Linguistic note – The word 'microbiome' is thought to be a portmanteau of 'microbiota' and 'genome'. The microbiota are the microbial flora harboured by individuals. Genome means the complete genetic information (either DNA or, in some viruses, RNA) of an organism. This means the 'microbiome' is the sum total of the genetic information in any individual's microbial flora.

The flora in a normal gut constitute an essential part of our defence against disease. Experimentally-induced absence of gut flora in mice results in serious infections and premature death. Our current epidemics of autoimmunity partly derive from our increasingly abnormal microbiomes.

The normal gut microbiome

The normal upper gut should be a near-sterile, digesting organ to deal with fat and protein. It is the lower gut, the colon, where microbes should flourish. In the healthy lower gut, there are about 14,000 different species of microbes, numbering about 100 trillion and weighing over a kilogram. Indeed, there are 10 times more microbes here than human cells in the body. We acquire microbes from our mother, who, we can only hope, has been eating a paleo-ketogenic diet (based on fat and fibre whole foods, not carbs) and has never received a course of antibiotics. Those microbes are picked up during vaginal delivery and nourished by breastmilk, which is full of the prebiotic inulin.

The naïve baby's immune system is like a computer that needs software – and it simply accepts as normal whatever is presented. Any deviation from the afore-stated perfection may result in a less than ideal inoculation and a less than ideal gut microbiome for life.

The gut flora is remarkably stable and unique, not just to that individual but also to different anatomical sites. The species of microbe on one tooth will be unique to that tooth and different from the adjacent tooth. The same is true of skin – the microbes on my index finger are unique to that and different from my thumb. As I type I deposit microbes on my keyboard in a way unique to me and as diagnostically sensitive as DNA profiling.

Keep it normal

After we are born and inoculated as described, the most important determinant of gut microbes is diet. Given the right substrate and conditions, microbes can double their number every 20 minutes. Given adverse conditions, they can go to sleep but wake at a moment's notice – they are great survivors. This makes our microbiome wonderfully robust. It remains stable through feast and famine. This works very much in our favour when the microbiome is friendly. By contrast, if it is less than friendly it is equally difficult to change for the better.

Many people imagine that to correct or improve the gut flora, or to protect ourselves from the disrupting effects of antibiotics, all we need to do is to swallow some probiotic capsules. The fact is these will be largely destroyed by stomach acid. Even those that survive the acid bath will have little hope of colonising the lining of the gut. It is a xenophobic issue – yes, microbes do not like outsiders. Those indigenous to the gut are already living in a crowded space and fighting for resources – they are not going to allow strangers into their midst. Indeed, this is a likely mechanism of protection against infections. Any strange microbes that evade stomach acid can be crowded out by the indigenous population.

Train the immune system

Having said that, we do know that taking probiotics does protect against infection – traveller's diarrhoea is a well-studied example. Post-weaning infectious diarrhoea is a particular problem in the pig industry and probiotics are of proven benefit. To stand the best chance of oral probiotics doing some good for the gut microbiome, they have to be live specimens taken in large amounts. But even dead microbes have beneficial effects. This means that the best results will come from cultured (that is, fermented) foods. I think of this as training the immune system – we also train human soldiers with dummies that can't fight back. That teaches recognition, respect and restraint.

There is a further reason why it is almost impossible to correct gut flora using probiotics. Roughly 90% of the gut flora is oxygen hating ('anaerobic') and will be killed by such. These microbes survive, indeed flourish, in the large bowel because the oxygen levels in the lumen of the colon are very low. Within a few minutes of defaecation these anaerobic microbes will be killed by air or go into hibernation. In practice, there are three possible mechanisms by which anaerobic microbes can be used to improve the gut microbiome from top down or bottom up:

1. good fresh local, dirty vegetables and sauerkraut (stalactites – i.e. top down);
2. 'faecal bacteriotherapy' (stalagmites – i.e. bottom up).

To remember the relevant orifices this jingle helps:

The mites go up and the tights come down.

Mr Jerry Rowe – Sarah's chemistry teacher circa 1975

Good fresh local dirty vegetables

We come from the earth, we return to the earth, and between the two we garden.
Maria Chaworth Musters, wonderful gardener and dear friend (1926 – 2010)

Humans evolved to be bred, born and reared in one locality. Not only did they learn to deal with the local soil microbes, but they also turned them to good advantage. Even in the case of nomadic populations, the soil types might have been more extensive, but these people were still exposed to 'known' soil microbes, in the sense their bodies had evolved to recognise these on the regular routes they took. It is an inevitable part of being a good gardener that hands are soiled and stained. I dig my roots, weed and pick vegetables with grimy hands. I may brush off the worst of the mud, but those same grubby paws prepare my food. This further helps to inoculate my gut with soil organisms. This process is further assisted by my faithful terrier Nancy who joins me at the table, shares my meat and licks up the spills, including the tasty crusty bits at the corners of my mouth. At a recent conference, I was delighted to watch a video clip of Consultant Immunologist Professor Yehuda Shoenfeld's dog licking his grand-daughter's head and neck – pure pleasure registered on all faces.

We know more about the movement of celestial bodies than about the soil underfoot.

Leonardo da Vinci, circa 1510

Note on celestial mechanics: We don't actually know as much about celestial mechanics as we would like to think either. The '*n*-body problem' is the problem of predicting the individual motions of a group of celestial objects interacting with each other gravitationally. There is no general exact solution to the *n*-body problem for $n > 2$ and we must rely on numerical methods and number crunching.

Sauerkraut

Sauerkraut is fermented by soil microbes that are naturally present on the leaves of the plants used. I would not dare presume which species from the 14,000 we know of are the important ones. Mimic nature. Use sauerkrauts that are made from vegetables, grown organically on healthy soils with live ferments and no additives. That is about as scientific as I can get! Details of how to prepare such can be found in our book *The PK Cookbook*. I have to say, I spend more time talking about food and cooking than all other subjects put together. If you choose to read just one other of our other books, go for *The PK Cookbook*. This will have the most profound effects on your health.

Editorial note – Craig is still trying his best to convert his wife, Penny, to a PK diet and is having some success. Wandering round the supermarket, and as Penny picks up items such as biscuits and cakes, Craig can be heard quoting Sarah – 'That looks like food, but it isn't!' or more recently, simply, 'Looks like food, isn't!'. Other shoppers look on aghast at this 'madman'!

Faecal bacteriotherapy

Faecal bacteriotherapy goes a step further. First the gut is emptied using a laxative such as Epsom salts. It is then colonised with fresh turds from a healthy human donor. Try to ignore the yuk factor and be grateful this is not a stalactite treatment! This is of proven benefit; indeed, it is the treatment of choice in ulcerative colitis, pseudomembranous colitis and *Clostridium difficile* infection. It has even been shown to be helpful in other conditions associated with abnormal microbiome, such as chronic fatigue syndrome, autism and Parkinson's disease. Interestingly, it is the *diversity* of microbes in the gut that is a marker of good health – the more species the better. My guess is that each gut microbe is food-specific, so the more varied your diet, the more varied your gut microbes. Furthermore, 15% of the microbiome is viral – not viruses that attack humans but viruses that attack bacteria. These are called bacteriophages ('bacteria eaters'). All ecosystems include predators, prey and parasites.

When the Iron Curtain divided East from West, researchers in the West developed antibiotics to treat bacterial infections, but researchers to the East developed phages. Where there are bacteria there are phages – indeed, on planet Earth they outnumber all bacteria. These viruses have huge untapped potential and are already used in the food industry to control Listeria contaminations. My guess is that by eating grubby vegetables and good sauerkraut we will be constantly re-inoculating our gut with bacteriophages.

The bacteriophages demonstrate that ancient proverb admirably:

The enemy of my enemy is my friend.

This phrase is first credited to the Indian philosopher Chanakya, or Kautilya, who wrote about the concept in Book VI, *The Source of Sovereign States* and lived in the 4th century BC.[30]

Chapter 9

Vitamin C – our most important weapon

What happens if a straight line doesn't get enough vitamin C?

It gets curvy

Groan! But now onto the serious stuff – and Vitamin C is very serious in our fight against infections.

Vitamin C is the most powerful, broad-spectrum antimicrobial that we have available to us. It is completely safe to human cells, with no known toxicity. It should be available for routine use in all cases of infectious disease and, arguably, in all pathology. Vitamin C has been forgotten simply because it cannot be patented by a drug company and no significant money can therefore be made from its sales; since the pharmaceutical companies now control medical brain-washing (whoops – I mean education), it has been written out of the curriculum.

> Hippocrates (460 – 370 BC) said, 'Of several remedies, the physician should choose the least sensational', which would amply describe the use of vitamin C. This may be one of the earliest examples of many similar thoughts on the virtues of simplicity. Sir Isaac Newton believed that Nature was pleased with simplicity and directed his mind to finding the least complicated solution to a particular problem that simultaneously solved all its facets. Once he had found such a solution, he stopped. The US Navy in the 1960s had a design principle for its engineers – the KISS Principle – 'Keep It Simple, Sweetheart'.

Vitamin C has been ignored by the medical profession for several reasons:

- The dose necessary to prevent scurvy is a tiny 30 milligrams (mg) per day. The ridiculous (whoops again – I mean, recommended) daily dose of vitamin C is therefore set at the 'let's stop scurvy' dose of between 40 and 100 mg daily. This is far too low for infection prevention and treatment.

- Because of the above, a dose of 500-1000 mg is described as high. This too is a nonsense. If we project from animals that can make their own vitamin C, then we should be taking at least 5000 mg (that is, 5 grams, or approximately a teaspoonful) of vitamin C daily. It is impossible to get this sort of amount from a Western diet. Many of my patients believe that fruit is an essential source of vitamin C, but the harmful effects of fruit sugar are not mitigated by any vitamin C that may be present. Fruit is a bag of sugar. Berries are the only fruit sufficiently low in sugar to be safe on a paleo-ketogenic diet.

- Humans are particularly susceptible to vitamin C deficiency because, alongside guinea pigs, fruit bats and dry-nosed primates, and by contrast with other mammals, they cannot make it themselves. When animals become ill they hugely ramp up their production of vitamin C – goats, for example, have been shown to produce 15,000 mg (that is, 15 grams) daily.

- When Westerners are given increasing doses of vitamin C they eventually get diarrhoea. This is known as the 'bowel tolerance' dose which varies for each of us. This is considered an unpleasant side effect and so people are advised not to take high doses because of it. Actually, this is a marvellous tool for treating the upper fermenting gut and killing unfriendly invaders. The starting point for treating all infection is to take vitamin C to bowel tolerance – see below.

- To achieve bowel tolerance, most normally-well people need 5000 to 15,000 mg (5–15 grams) daily. However, where there is infection anywhere in the body the bowel tolerance increases hugely – for some, up to 200 grams per day. Flip this logic and one can see that the bowel tolerance of vitamin C is an indirect test of the total infectious load of the body, which may be local to the fermenting gut or systemic. This is a very useful clinical tool because one does not even have to diagnose which infection is present nor tailor a specific treatment since vitamin C does it for all. I have to say, I do like inexpensive, safe, quick, DIY medical diagnostic and therapeutic tools!

- As a result of the above ignorance of the basic properties of vitamin C, the doses used in any study or trial have been far too low. Had antibiotics been subject to the same level of under-dosing they too would never have been developed.

No evidence compels the conclusion that the minimum required intake of any vitamin comes close to the optimum intake that sustains good health.
Linus Pauling (1901 – 1994), advocate of vitamin C in large doses and one of the greatest scientists of all time. He was the only ever winner of two Nobel Prizes (unshared). He was only just beaten to a third by Watson and Crick.

There is a fascinating relationship between vitamin C and sugar (glucose) which has yet to be fully elucidated. I think vitamin C and sugar are two sides of the same coin: they are physically similar molecules – indeed, in most mammals, vitamin C is made from sugar in a four-enzyme step process. Pretty much all the conditions that sugar makes worse, including hypertension, diabetes, cancer, dementia, arterial disease and heart disease, vitamin C protects against. In the gut, vitamin C and sugar compete for absorption. This is bad news – Western diets, being high in sugar, therefore increase the risk of vitamin C deficiency. By 'deficiency' in humans, I mean being below the dose of vitamin C necessary for optimum health. So, Westerners are more deficient in vitamin C (owing to their diets) and therefore need higher doses for optimum health. Vitamin C and sugar also compete for absorption in bacteria, yeasts and cancer cells. Starve these cells of sugar, feed them with vitamin C instead, and you kill them. There we have our mantra again – starve and kill to win the infection game.

We know vitamin C is directly toxic to bacteria and yeast because it is widely used as a food preservative. Frederick R Klenner tells us that 'vitamin C takes up the protein coats being manufactured by the virus nucleic acid, thus preventing the assembly of new virus units. Cells expand, rupture and die, but there are no virus particles available to enter and infect new cells. If a virus has invaded a cell, the vitamin C contributes to its breakdown through adenosine deaminase, which converts adenosine to inosine. Purines are formed which are catabolized (broken down) and cannot be used to make more virus nucleic acid.'[31] (see Chapter 4)

Regardless, I do know that vitamin C used in high doses regularly, and in super-high doses at the first sign of any cough, cold or influenza, is highly effective in preventing the illness from developing or progressing. It kills viruses on contact. It is essential to the immune system to kill microbes – it is part of the immune system's ammunition and is an extraordinary weapon because its use does not result in friendly-fire damage. Indeed, it helps to mitigate this. The immune system's need for vitamin C increases hugely with infection and, as I have said, this is reflected by the dose necessary to cause diarrhoea – such 'bowel tolerance' vitamin C doses increase markedly during periods of infection.

So, taking super-high doses of vitamin C during an infection:

- directly kills all microbes on contact;
- mitigates any friendly-fire damage by the immune system;
- mops up the free radicals inevitably produced as energy delivery mechanisms are increased.

Vitamin C must be used early on during the onset of an infection and in high doses. Hit your enemy soon and hit him hard! Indeed, the single greatest reason for vitamin C failure is that not a large enough dose has been used. By taking large doses by mouth to cause diarrhoea one sweeps the invaders out of the gut before they can get a foothold on *terra firma* and any that have got into the body are killed. Reduce the number of invaders and you make the immune system army mega-sized by comparison. As Dr Klenner said:

The patient should get large doses of vitamin C in all pathological conditions while the physician ponders the diagnosis.

Dr Frederick Robert Klenner, BS MS MD FCCP FAAFP (1907 – 1984)

From 1943 through 1947, Klenner reported successful treatment of 42 cases of viral pneumonia using therapeutic doses of vitamin C. This was administered by mouth, intravenously and intramuscularly.[32]

He subsequently used therapeutic doses of vitamin C as above to cure hundreds of cases of infection, including polio, Rocky Mountain fever, pneumonia and other such infectious diseases. He stated:

We've used massive doses of vitamins on over 10,000 people over a period of 30 years, and we've never seen any ill effects from them. The only effects we've seen have been beneficial.[33]

Editorial note: However, see the note below (page 60) about glucose-6-phosphate dehydrogenase deficiency and injected vitamin C.

The practical details

On a regular basis:

- Do the PK (paleo-ketogenic) diet – vitamin C is much better absorbed in the absence of sugar and starch. There is no point killing microbes with vitamin C if you are feeding them at the same time.
- Take ascorbic acid (see below) at least twice daily (and it could be more often – in severe infections it should be every hour). It dissolves much better in warm water. Add fizzy water to produce a rather delicious drink! Remember, ascorbic acid is an acid so rinse your mouth with water after drinking it to protect your tooth enamel. The ascorbic acid helps to sterilise the upper gut and prevents fermentation of food. Any microbes inadvertently consumed with foods are killed. Acid further helps digest proteins and the absorption of essential minerals such as iron and zinc.
- Use ascorbic acid, which is the cheapest and most effective form of vitamin C. If this is not tolerated, then use a neutral preparation, such as sodium or magnesium ascorbate. Once you are PK- and vitamin C-adapted, you should tolerate ascorbic acid well. The cheapest form of ascorbic acid is fermented from corn but if you are allergic to the corn you may not tolerate this at all, in which case you can get ascorbic acid from sago palm. (Nutri-West produce a sago-based vitamin C that is available from www.pureformulas.com)
- Start with 2 grams twice daily (4 grams in total) and increase at the rate of 1 gram every day. You will start to get foul-smelling wind. This occurs because microbes in the upper gut are being killed, swept downstream and fermented by microbes in the lower gut. This is likely to need more than 10 grams of vitamin C. Keep increasing the dose until you get diarrhoea. Hold the dose at this level for 24 hours. At this point you should have a clean, digesting (non-fermenting) upper gut with low levels of microbes in the lower gut.
- Adjust the daily dose in the longer term. The idea is to find a dose of vitamin C that kills the grams of unfriendly microbes in the upper gut but does not kill the kilograms of friendly microbes in the lower gut. This will depend on several variables that you will have to work out for yourself, vis:
  - o   A dose that allows you to pass a normally formed daily turd
  - o   No smelly farting

o   A dose that stops you getting coughs, colds and 'flu when all around are succumbing

o   A dose that reduces, gets rid of or reverses any disease symptoms that you may be suffering from. These may be symptoms of the upper fermenting gut (burping, discomfort, reflux) or of chronic infection. As you will see from the Cathcart link below, you have to get to 80-90% of bowel tolerance to reverse the symptoms of any disease process.

At the first hint of any infection, such as a tickle in the throat, runny nose, sneeze, cough, feeling unwell, headache, cystitis... well, you know what from bitter experience:

- immediately take 10 grams of vitamin C. If this does not produce diarrhoea within one hour
- take another 10 grams. If this does not produce diarrhoea within one hour
- take another 10 grams... and so on. Some people need 200 grams to get a result. Whilst this may seem like a huge dose, compare this with sugar – four bars of milk chocolate would provide a similar dose of sugar, and vitamin C is legions safer than sugar.
- Some people are appalled at the idea of vitamin C causing diarrhoea, but I have to say I would rather have a jolly good bowel emptying crap than suffer the miserable symptoms of 'flu or a cold for the next two weeks. Indeed, I have not suffered from such for 35 years thanks to vitamin C. My father used to say, 'You can't beat a good shit, shave and shampoo.'
- Adjust the frequency and timing of subsequent doses to maintain wellness.
- Remember, the dose is critical. You cannot overdose, you can only under-dose. Just do it!

I am not alone in this advice. Dr Robert Cathcart was a similar advocate of high-dose vitamin C.[34] Key points in this paper (https://vitamincfoundation.org/www.orthomed. com/titrate.htm) are:

- Everyone's bowel tolerance dose is unique to them. It will vary through time with age, diet and infectious load. You have to work it out for yourself and it will not remain constant.
- You must get to 80-90% of your bowel tolerance dose for vitamin C to relieve

symptoms. This is another useful clinical tool as you can feel so much better so very quickly if you use vitamin C properly.

Cathcart details many diseases that are improved with vitamin C. Interestingly, this includes many cases of arthritis. I suspect this illustrates one mechanism of arthritis which is that it is often driven by allergy to gut microbes. Correct this and the arthritis goes. For example, we know ankylosing spondylitis is an inflammation driven by *Klebsiella* in the gut and rheumatoid arthritis is driven by *Proteus mirabilis*.

Dr Paul Marik from the Eastern Virginia Medical School in Norfolk, Virginia, added intravenous vitamin C to his normal antibiotic protocol for treating patients diagnosed with advanced sepsis and septic shock in his intensive care unit. Before using vitamin C the mortality was 40%. Mortality is now less than 1%. Had this been a novel antibiotic it would have made headline news.

Dr Marik offered the following observations:

In the doses used, vitamin C is absolutely safe. No complications, side effects or precautions. Patients with cancer have safely been given doses up to 150 grams – one hundred times the dose we give. In the patients with renal impairment we have measured the oxalate levels; these have all been in the safe range. Every single patient who received the protocol had an improvement in renal function.[35, 36]

It is important to be aware that anyone receiving *intravenous* vitamin C must be first checked for glucose-6-phosphate dehydrogenase (G6P) deficiency. High-dose vitamin C in these people may cause haemolytic anaemia (a form of anaemia due to haemolysis – the abnormal breakdown of red blood cells, either in the blood vessels (intravascular haemolysis) or elsewhere in the human body (extravascular), but usually in the spleen). I can find no evidence of this being an issue for oral vitamin C.

Lots more good science and practical detail can be found at 'AscorbateWeb': http://seanet.com/~alexs/ascorbate/index.htm#Rev-Ed. And if nothing else, please do remember that vitamin 'C' is Spanish for vitamin 'Yes'!

Chapter 10

Iodine – a great all-rounder

Iodine kills all classes of pathogen on contact: viruses, bacteria, fungi, yeasts and protozoa. Most bacteria are killed within 30 seconds of contact. The mechanism is that iodine kills single-celled organisms by combining with the amino acids tyrosine or histidine. All single-celled organisms showing tyrosine on their outer cell membranes are killed instantly by a simple chemical reaction with iodine that denatures proteins. No microbe is resistant. Selvaggi et al in 2003 concluded that the antibacterial effect of iodine was superior to that of other products and that, unlike antibiotics and other antiseptics, it seemed to have no resistance problems.[37]

Interestingly, iodine is also very safe to take by mouth. The French physician Lugol in 1829 developed Lugol's iodine, which was a mixture of 5% iodine with 10% potassium iodide, which greatly enhanced the absorption of iodine. He prescribed 300 to 1000 mg (Lugol's 12% iodine 40 to 160 drops, 2 to 8 ml) per day for the treatment of infectious disease, with good results. This shows how safe iodine is to take internally. Not only is this helpful in reducing microbial numbers by contact kill, but iodine is also an essential part of good immune function. To quote Dr David Derry:

> *Extremely high doses of iodine can have serious side effects, but only a small fraction of such extreme doses are necessary to kill influenza viruses. In 1945, a breakthrough occurred when J.D. Stone and Sir McFarland Burnet (who later went on to win a Nobel Prize for his clonal selection theory) exposed mice to lethal effects of influenza viral mists. The lethal disease was prevented by putting iodine solution on mice snouts just prior to placing them in chambers containing influenza viruses.*[38]

Iodine is by far the best antibiotic, antiviral and antiseptic of all time.[39]

Your daily dose of iodine

What the daily dose of iodine should be is debatable, but, like vitamin C, what we do know is that the daily need for iodine is far higher than the 'recommended daily amount' (RDA), which is set at a risible 150 micrograms (mcg). This takes no account of iodine deficiency, which is pandemic in Western society. Deficiency is compounded by the increasing use of competing halides, such as fluoride (water, toothpaste, dental treatments and many drugs, especially slow-release drugs) and bromide (polybrominated biphenyls or PBBs used as fire retardants in soft furnishings, and chocolate, which is high in bromide).

At the very least, one should use Sunshine salt (see page 238) which contains 1 mg of iodine per teaspoon and will prevent overt deficiency. However, if there is any doubt, then test as follows.

Test for iodine sufficiency – do you have enough?

The best test is to measure urine iodine excretion. However, a clinical test that may give some idea is a simple skin test. Use Lugol's 12% 4 drops to paint a patch on your inner forearm about 10 x 10 cm. This will stain the skin dark yellow. Allow it to dry. Observe. As much as 24 hours later you should be able to see the stain. If not, that suggests iodine deficiency.

If you are deficient, then repletion may take some weeks of taking a loading dose. I suggest 25 mg daily (that is, two Iodoral 12.5 mg tablets daily (see page 219) or 4 drops of Lugol's iodine 12%). Once replete, my view is that one should take 25 mg weekly to maintain sufficient levels. Iodine is not only an excellent antimicrobial but also effective at stripping out toxic metals. (I have never done a test of toxic metals and not found any.) Iodine helps to mitigate increasing environmental pollution and to combat the increasing infection risks of modern life. This regime is very safe.

Iodine to treat surface infections and respiratory infections

There is a happy synergy with vitamin C. Remember, the more different ways one can hit microbes the better. Iodine should be applied *ad lib* externally. It is volatile and penetrates the skin well. Combine this with vitamin C internally and one gets a classic pincer movement so beloved of army generals. I also liken it to Muhammed Ali … a right hook of vitamin C followed by an iodine left upper cut takes no prisoners! To be effective you need a decent dose. The key is in the colour – iodine stains tissues yellow; when the yellow is gone so is the iodine. Reapply.

Table 10.1: How to use iodine to best effect

Problem	Use	Notes
Skin	Iodine ointment 10% is ideal for all skin breaches, burns, cuts, ulcers, spots, boils, warts and verrucas.	Use *ad lib* – the skin should be permanently stained yellow with iodine. It is volatile so penetrates deep into the skin. It kills on contact but is completely non-toxic to the healing process.
Fungal infections	Athlete's foot Tinea of the groin or armpit Balanitis Dandruff or cradle cap of the scalp	You have to use it regularly to be effective. Initially the scalp will stain yellow but it evaporates and goes – then reapply
Crusty eyelashes	Usually a fungal infection – iodine ointment 10%	Use *ad lib*
Shingles, chicken pox, hand and mouth	Use *ad lib* to greatly reduce the infectious load	Also take vitamin C to bowel tolerance. See Chapter 17 – Groundhog Acute (page 110)
Cold sores	Ditto above	Ditto
Recurrent nose bleeds or inflammation	Smear iodine ointment inside the nose and on the skin round the outside of the nose	These are often due to *Staphylococcus aureus* in the nose – indeed, MRSA may be carried in the nose. This will also protect you from inhaled virus and may be very useful in the event of a 'flu epidemic

Problem	Use	Notes
All eye infections: conjunctivitis, iritis	Povodine-iodine eye drops 5% *ad lib* OR 2 drops of Lugol's iodine 12% in 5 ml of water does not sting the eyes and is the best killer of all microbes in the eye	Again, iodine penetrates well. Use *ad lib* at least four times daily. There is evidence that many degenerative eye conditions are driven by infection, including macular degeneration
		Iodine is also a very good treatment for dry eyes
Ear infections of external canal	Put a dollop of iodine ointment 10% in the opening of your ear canal, then lie down on your side so the iodine melts and runs in to your ear canal	This may also help otitis media since iodine is volatile and penetrates well
Boils, acne, impetigo	Use *ad lib* on and around the area of infection	Combine with vitamin C to bowel tolerance (see Chapter 9)
Paronychia (nail-bed infection)	Ditto	The key is to keep the skin stained yellow with iodine
Ulcers and bedsores	Ditto	Combine with vitamin C to bowel tolerance. Leg ulcers need proper pressure graduated hosiery to ensure good blood flow. I recommend Daylong (see page 218)
Mouth ulcers, gingivitis, pharyngitis, tonsillitis	Take Lugol's iodine 12% 4 drops in a small glass of water every hour OR chew iodoral 12.5 mg – hold in the mouth as long as possible at least four times daily	Safe to swallow.
Respiratory infections	Use a salt pipe – put 4 drops of Lugol's iodine 12% into the chamber (this can be easily done through the 'air out' end of the salt chamber). Salt is of proven additional benefit	Use this inhalation at least four times a day to contact-kill all pathogens in the mouth, nose, throat and air passages of the bronchi and lungs. This often works remarkably well for people with chronic lung infections, such as bronchiectasis

64

Fungal toenails	Apply iodine as often as necessary to keep the affected nails stained yellow	
Anal fissure, piles	Use iodine ointment *ad lib*	
Genital sores or warts	Ditto	

I have often wondered why it is that many of the body's lymph nodes are so superficial, such as those in the neck, elbow creases, armpits, back of the knees and groin. It may be that the body holds microbes here so they can be destroyed by the light of sunshine penetrating the skin. My guess is that iodine would be equally efficient, and I suggest applying iodine ointment *ad lib* over any tender lymph nodes. Being volatile it penetrates the flesh well to contact kill.

> When I was a medical student, iodine in the form of KI [potassium iodide] was the universal medicine. Nobody knew what it did, but it did something and did something good. We students used to sum up the situation in this little rhyme: 'If you do not know where, what and why, prescribe ye then K and I.'
>
> Albert Szent-Gyorgyi, Nobel Prize winner for medicine 1937
> who discovered vitamin C in 1928 (1893 – 1986)

Iodine and thyroid disease

Anyone with any thyroid problem should be taking iodine as above. However, when you first try iodine it is important to start at a low dose and build up slowly. This is because hypothyroidism is so common owing to iodine deficiency. When suddenly it appears in abundance the thyroid is driven to a temporary state of overproduction.

Be aware that falling intakes of iodine in the diet over recent years have been paralleled by a huge increase in hypothyroidism, thyrotoxicosis and autoimmune thyroid disease.

Allergy to iodine is possible

The immune system in the skin is different from that in the mouth and gut – it may be that if you react allergically in one department you can be tolerant in another. Iodine is well absorbed through the skin, so if oral supplements are not possible then use Lugol's drops undiluted and directly onto the skin. Approximately 12% is absorbed (the rest evaporates) – that is, you need 8 drops of Lugol's 12% on the skin to achieve a similar oral dose of one drop.

The Wolff-Chaikoff effect

This effect is a reduction in thyroid hormone levels caused by ingestion of a large amount of iodine. It is a protective mechanism against iodine overdose whereby the blood supply to the thyroid gland is temporarily reduced and in consequence so is the output of thyroid hormones. This is very useful for:

- treating a 'thyroid storm' in acute thyrotoxicosis
- using before surgery to minimise bleeding
- inhibiting uptake of radioactive iodine in the event of a nuclear accident with exposure to such.

Guy E Abraham has written a fascinating history of the use of iodine in medicine.[40] In this he concludes that there were many monographs attesting to iodine's efficacy written in the early 1800s but that only recently has iodine been rediscovered as a universal medicine.

Historical note: Jean Lugol was a French physician. He was a fascinating man and the article by E Neuzil in 2002[41] describes him thus:

…an excellent practitioner who constantly proved a great independence of spirit towards some medical concepts 'à la mode' … very close to his patients… who admired… the efficiency of his therapeutic innovations, his intellectual uprightness.

Note from Craig: This sounds very much like a female British physician of modern times to me…
Note from Sarah: I can see why Penny fell for him!

Chapter 11

Electromagnetic radiation:
the good (heat and light) and
the bad (electro-smog)

Running a fever is an excellent way of killing microbes, but it is metabolically expensive, which is why the immune system reserves this for serious infections. Interestingly, running a fever is accompanied by the sensation of feeling cold. This symptom is so uncomfortable it makes us swing into action, wrap up warm, curl up next to a good fire and slurp hot drinks – a perfect behavioural response. The brain is helping the immune system fight and sweat out the infection.

Many people swear by a hot sauna or a hot bath to cure acute infection. The logic is clear to see. What I do not advocate is exercising to generate heat and a fever. If you are lucky this will work, but if energy delivery mechanisms are on the edge, then intense exercise will take essential energy resources away from the immune system, rendering it less capable. Indeed, I have many patients whose CFS was triggered by infection combined with a misguided attempt to 'run it off'.

Dr Friedrich Douwes MD reckons that hyperthermia increases the effectiveness of antibiotics (by a factor of 60-fold!) and kills microbes, including Lyme, directly. Moreover, research in 1996 showed that 10% of *Borrelia* bacteria were killed when exposed to this temperature.[42] Douwes uses a large incubator to increase the body temperature over two hours to 41.6°Celsius (107°F), holds it there for two hours, and then slowly reduces it over a further two hours. He reckons to cure 60% of Lyme cases with this method. He has shown hyperthermia to be effective against all the herpes viruses. My guess is hyperthermia will be effective against many infections.

Before the advent of antibiotics, malaria therapy was used to treat syphilis. The idea here was that malaria induced a great fever and this killed the *Treponema pallidum* spirochete (a particular class of bacterium) responsible for syphilis. This worked well for some, but an unfortunate side effect was that others died of malaria. Perhaps that was more socially acceptable? Heat therapy is also a recognised treatment for cancer. It may be that cancer cells are more susceptible to heat, but since many cancers are driven by infection it may be that heat is working via a microbe-killing action.

The attraction of hyperthermia to treat infection is high because this is a tool we can all easily employ. The key is to measure core temperature to make sure you do not (literally) cook. The *Guinness Book of Records* no longer holds details of heat tolerant competitions because people have died in their attempts to win. Be mindful that a high fever, particularly in children, can cause seizures. Whilst these are frightening they are remarkably harmless and easily treated by cooling. They rarely occur with core temperatures up to 40°C but this sort of temperature is still highly effective at killing microbes.

Light therapy

To the Ancient Greeks and Romans, the sun was Apollo's fiery chariot making its way across the sky, bringing life-giving light to the planet. Apollo was the god of medicine and healing as well as of sun and light. Frequently, in the Ancient world, healing was associated with warmth, light *and* 'Nature'. Indeed, the Romans, like our mothers, understood only too well that:

> medicus curat, natura sanat – *idiomatic translation: 'The doctor cares [or should do!], and Nature heals'.*
>
> Old Latin Proverb, Proverb 1087, 4000 in *Latin via Proverbs*
> by Laura Gibb

The chapters and advice in this book are partly about allowing Nature the space to do this healing herself and where necessary giving a helping hand. This 'helping hand' is needed because modern Western lifestyles have often changed the goalposts for Nature, so we must intervene to redress the natural state of affairs.

Ultraviolet (UV) light kills all microbes. How do I know that? It is already used to sterilise water for drinking and swimming pools. Sunshine was the main treatment for tuberculosis (TB) in the pre-antibiotic era. On the London Science Museum's website it states that in the late 1800s heliotherapy became a treatment for tuberculosis as exposure to sunlight killed bacteria. Many of the patients were children from city slums; the increased exposure to sunlight also raised their vitamin D levels, which additionally helped them to fight the infection. The website also goes on to explain that Niels Ryberg Finsen won the Nobel Prize in 1903 for his Finsen Lamp, an ultraviolet lamp that allowed such treatments throughout all seasons and could also be concentrated on the most affected part of the patient's body.[43]

Light as a treatment for infection has been used for years for serious infections. In one technique, the patient receives treatment by removing a pint of blood, irradiating it with light, then returning it to the body. The problem with this treatment is that it is high tech and expensive. However, equally good results can be obtained by intranasal light. This makes perfect sense – the nasal mucosa is thin and so light can easily get to the bloodstream. The nose is well perfused with blood and so it is easily radiated. But most importantly the results obtained with intranasal light are as good as with intravenous treatment. Indeed, it may be that intranasal light impacts directly on the brain and this could be helpful for any patient with brain pathology.[44]

As you will see from the pictures and videos on www.mediclights.com, light restores normal circulation by unclogging red blood cells, making them less sticky. It is also worth one minute and fifty seconds to look at this YouTube clip (www.youtube.com/watch?v=nfUQNJWDFqQ) entitled 'Vielight – Blood Disaggregation Video', 'disaggregation' being another way of saying 'making less sticky'. These results are obtained after just 25 minutes of light therapy. My guess is that the relevant red blood cells are sticky because of the presence of microbes in the blood; the idea here is that light kills these microbes and that this is reflected by a reduction in the stickiness of the blood.

The Vielight device (or Bionase)

The device that supplies this light can be seen at http://vielight.com/product/vielight-633/. Ten million have been sold, mostly in Russia and China. The conditions for which there is an excellent evidence base for positive responses include high blood pressure, high LDL cholesterol, diabetes, atherosclerosis, asthma, stroke, cancer, immune system deficiencies, infections, rheumatoid arthritis, fibromyalgia and psoriasis. All these conditions can be partly explained by fermenting gut and allergy/infection to microbes spilling over from the gut.

This device uses near-infrared light; interestingly there is some evidence that this 'kick starts' mitochondria to produce more ATP – the energy molecule.[45] This would also be helpful by improving energy delivery to the immune system to help it fight infection. This may be especially helpful for people with chronic sinus infections.

Sunbathing – heat and light

Sunshine is a delicious combination of heat and light. Both penetrate the skin and kill microbes, thereby reducing the infectious burden on our skin (great treatment for acne and eczema) and in the body. This means we spend less energy on the immune system, leaving more energy for other things. There is evidence that full-spectrum light may improve mitochondrial function. I have to say I don't really care about the scientific explanation – I just know I feel better for sunbathing!

I have many patients who feel well and recover simply by moving to a warm, sunny climate. Take any opportunity to sunbathe. You do need direct sunshine on the skin because glass will block ultraviolet light. So do sun tan lotions – do not use them! Sunbathe enough to brown not burn – with time you can tolerate much more sunshine. Indeed, there is evidence that suntan lotions, which are full of toxic chemicals, *increase* the risk of skin cancer.

TB sufferers treated with sunshine could not immediately tolerate full body exposure. Special trolleys were designed which could be pushed out onto balconies so initially just the feet were exposed, then legs, trunk and finally the whole body. Too much sun too soon made them ill. I wonder if this may be a Herxheimer reaction? (A Herxheimer reaction occurs when microbes are killed and there is an allergic reaction to the dead microbial detritus.) Indeed, Dr Horowitz comments that 50% of his Lyme patients were intolerant of sunshine and again I wonder if this too is a Herxheimer reaction? Doxycycline, often used to treat Lyme disease, can cause light sensitivity – again perhaps the mechanism of this is a Herx reaction? The important message here is not to be put off using light should such a reaction occur – it may be a good sign and may well pass with time. In the short term, reduce the dose of light; once tolerated, increase it again.

The Ancients knew the benefits of sunbathing and even had a verb for it – *apricari* (to bask in the sunshine). This gives us one of the great unused words in the English language – to apricate, meaning to bask in the sunshine. (For readers interested in unused words in the English language, the website www.unusedwords.com comes highly recommended by Craig.) Returning to Old Latin Proverb of 1087 (above), we can see that sunbathing is 'Nature' whereas the Vielight is a 'helping hand' – you will see that much of the advice in this book can be divided in this way. Go apricate!

Finally, some electromagnetic radiation is dangerous to health

First we had radiation… and they said that was safe. Then we had smoking… and it took 50 years for its toxicity to be accepted. Now we have electro-smog… and the electronic industry is even bigger than the tobacco industry. However, the epidemiology is fast catching up. It started with the observation of more Alzheimer's disease in poorly populated areas… why? In the early days of mobile phones, people living offline relied on them. The areas with the fastest rate of increase of Alzheimer's are developing areas.

Where the environment is so contaminated with this microwave pollution, insect numbers are down by 80% and song birds by 75%. Electro-smog has also been implicated in the aetiology of autism, and this together with toxic metals and opportunistic infections makes for a perfect neurological storm. It has been estimated that by 2025 50% of Western four-year-olds will be on the autistic spectrum.

It is biologically plausible that electromagnetic radiation is toxic for two reasons. It generates electrical fields in the body which will inevitably disrupt communication between cells and organs. Microwave radiation which is used for mobile and cordless phones and wifi generates heat. Indeed, that is how a microwave oven works. On YouTube you can see a video of mobile phones being used to cook an egg[46] and another using a mobile phone to cook popcorn.[47] I have recently heard of two cases of brain tumours which were situated immediately underneath where a blue tooth phone ear piece sat permanently.

Electromagnetic (EM) radiation may produce instant symptoms, such as headache or fatigue. This is called electrical sensitivity (ES) and for many is debilitating. Thanks to Professor Martin Pall we have a biochemical explanation for ES. EMF disrupts voltage-gated calcium channels across cell membranes. In a susceptible individual, ES will allow calcium to leak into cells (calcium is toxic inside cells – the normal concentration gradient of calcium outside to inside is a 14,000-fold difference). Since all cells have voltage-gated calcium channels, ES can present with any symptom.[48] So, what should we do?

- Diagnose
  - by using an electro-smog detector. This can be hired for short-term use from Healthy House (see page 218).
- Treat
  - by avoiding, or at least limiting, exposure to the worst offenders: mobile and cordless phones, wifi routers and smart meters;
  - by using blocking materials on the Faraday cage principle (again, see Recommended products on page 218.) (A Faraday cage is an enclosure used to block electromagnetic fields. A Faraday shield is made from a continuous covering of conductive material. A Faraday cage is made by forming a mesh of such materials. Faraday cages are named after the English scientist Michael Faraday, who invented them in 1836.)

Chapter 12

Dentists, doctors and other foreign bodies

Not many Westerners lack a foreign body. I have dental fillings and a length of metal which pins my fractured collar bone. A patient who consulted with me recently considered that earrings, tattoos and an IUCD (intra-uterine contraceptive device) to be the normal accoutrements of modern life, but those too are foreign bodies. I have been consulted by over 200 women with health problems following silicone breast implants.

> There is that great moment in the original *Planet of the Apes* film (1968) where Taylor (Charlton Heston) realises that he is in fact on 'his' Earth, looking at a 'modern' human skeleton, when he finds a pacemaker lying amongst the bones.

The body *is* xenophobic, hating foreigners, and does its best to get rid of them. This is a natural reaction to injuries involving foreign bodies, such as splinters of wood. These foreign bodies cause problems for at least three reasons:

1. They encourage infections because microbes can hide away inside them; this is akin to providing homes for terrorists. We have a particular problem with root canal fillings – microbes from the fermenting mouth easily slip between the gum and the tooth and can become entrenched in the root. If numbers build up suddenly, an abscess may result. However, the more pernicious issue seems to be the chronic leakage of microbes into the bloodstream which have the potential to drive inflammation at distal sites. Surgical implants may cause similar problems.

Indeed, we know that foreign bodies in bone are a risk for osteomyelitis. Silicone implants are often infected with fungi, such as *Aspergillus*; these are known to produce 'mycotoxins' (fungal poisons), such as ocratoxin – one probable cause of chronic fatigue syndrome/myalgic encephalitis (CFS/ME). It is almost impossible to get rid of a chronic uterine (womb) infection with an IUCD present.

2. Some foreign bodies contain materials which are toxic. In order of priority, these are mercury from dental amalgam, and nickel from piercings (nickel is a carcinogen) and bare-metal surgical stents. Although stenting of arteries seemed like a good idea at the time for the treatment of narrowed arteries to the heart, they often get blocked; why? Because the immune system is activated and the resulting inflammation blocks the artery completely. Meanwhile, the NHS is currently replacing 60,000 metal-on-metal hip replacements because of the toxicity of the stainless steel used.

3. Some foreign bodies contain materials which are immuno-toxic – that is to say, they switch on the immune system to drive allergy and autoimmunity. In order of priority, these are probably mercury from dental amalgam and silicone from silicone implants, the commonest use of which is in breast implants, but silicone is a widely used material in surgery, including hernia repairs, pacemakers, some slow-release implants such as contraceptives, shunt materials and testicular implants.

Prevention is the obvious tactic but people consult me when they are ill. In order of priority, the issues I think about are shown in Table 12.1.

Table 12.1: Potentially toxic foreign bodies

Material	Toxic?	Immuno-toxic?	Harbour microbes?	Notes
Dental amalgam (includes mercury, silver, tin, cadmium, lead, antimony, copper and zinc)	Yes	Yes	No – mercury kills microbes with the same efficiency that it kills human cells	Mercury is the most toxic element known to man apart from the radioactive elements. It leaks out of amalgam from the day it is inserted. No-one should be carrying any dental amalgam or, indeed, any metals in their mouth (see below)
Silicone, e.g. breast implants, testicular implants, mesh for hernia repair, tubes and pipes, body contouring; contraceptive implants	No	Yes	Yes	Again, silicone leaks out of implants from the day they are inserted. This drives autoimmune conditions, such as lupus erythematosus and multiple sclerosis. It is known that 50% rupture after 12 years and this accelerates the immuno-toxicity.*

*Table footnote: In fact leakage of silicone could be worse than that: Dr Edward Melmed, a plastic surgeon from Dallas, told an FDA (the US's Food & Drug Agency) panel that by 10 years after patients get them, 50% of silicone implants have ruptured, by 15 years, 72% and by 20 years, 94%. Meanwhile the US's Institute of Medicine has reported that 'Prevalence of rupture differing by brand of implant has been reported by Feng (IOM Scientific Workshop, 1998), and Peters and Francel have reported major differences in rupture for silicone gel implants of different vintages, up to 95% at 12 years' implantation with thin shelled, 1972-mid 1980s-implants (Francel et al., 1998; Peters et al., 1996).'[50, 51] A new syndrome – autoimmune/inflammatory syndrome induced by adjuvants (ASIA), which includes post-vaccination phenomena, macrophagic myofasciitis, Gulf War syndrome and siliconosis – has recently been described. This syndrome is characterised by non-specific and specific manifestations of autoimmune disease. Interested readers are directed to the study by Colaris et al (2017).[52]

Material	Toxic?	Immuno-toxic?	Harbour microbes?	Notes
Root canals	No	Possibly	Yes	Ecomed doctors (doctors who belong to the British Society of Ecological Medicine – www.bsem.org.uk) have seen many cases of CFS/ME, arthritis and autoimmunity resolve when root canals are dealt with by a knowledgeable dentist
Piercings	Yes	Yes	Yes	At least these are easy to get rid of!
Braces, wires, mixed metals in the mouth	Probably. When two different metals are in contact in the wet environment of the mouth there is a 'small battery' effect which increases the release of metals into the saliva	Indirectly	No	Metals in the mouth dissolve in saliva and are swallowed. Where there is a fermenting gut, hydrogen sulphide may be produced. This may convert an insoluble inorganic metal into a soluble organic metal which is much better absorbed and consequently bio-accumulates in the body – typically in the heart, brain, bone marrow and kidneys
Other dental materials, e.g. palladium, titanium, gold, platinum, cobalt, stainless steel, chromium, nickel		Some people sensitise to metals – there is the potential to be allergic to any dental metal		Cripes – these dentists have much to answer for! As a child my teeth were trencher-filled on the grounds that 'Darling, the fillings will be stronger than your teeth.' Perhaps, but I do not wish to be the corpse with the strongest teeth in the morgue

Nickel	Yes	Yes	Like mercury this is toxic to microbes	The toxicity of nickel is greatly under-rated. It is a known carcinogen
Surgical metal work: plates, rods and screws	Yes	Possibly	Yes	Bone infections are almost impossible to clear with antibiotics when a foreign material is present
Bare-metal stents for arteries	Possibly	Yes	Yes	All stents – bare metal, plastic and eluting – have problems. The jury is still out as to which material performs best
Tattoos: titanium, aluminium, toxic dyes	Yes	Yes	Possibly – see Note below	My naughty daughters once tricked me by appearing with a large tattoo each. As they watched me start to explode and become dangerous they realised their predicament and quickly admitted it was a temporary job…

If prevention is not possible, then:

- If safe and possible, remove the foreign body – such as dental amalgam, breast implants. This must be done safely.
- But remember some foreign bodies, such as my metal pin, may be impossible to get rid of and we are stuck with them.
- If removal is not safe or possible, then follow the advice in this book to mitigate the effects.

Note: In 2012, there was a small outbreak of skin infections in upstate New York. The source of the infections was traced back to a batch of grey ink that had been contaminated with bacteria called mycobacteria – cases as reported by Dr Marie Leger, a dermatologist at the New York University Langone Medical Center.[53]

Chapter 13

Herbals: delicious doctoring
They too fight the arms race and can help us

Winston Churchill made reference to the need to use whatever allies you can find when in the heat of war:

> *If Hitler invaded hell I would make at least a favourable reference to the devil in the House of Commons.*

Sir Winston Leonard Spencer Churchill, KG OM CH TD PC DL FRS RA

(30 November 1874 – 24 January 1965)

Fortunately for us, we do not have to make Faustian pacts but instead can find allies amongst plants and fungi.

Plants and fungi have been similarly involved in the arms race even longer than mammals. They too are survivors and have evolved equally intelligent and effective strategies to fight off microbial attack. We can jump on their band wagon by eating them. There is a massive scientific literature detailing the benefits of plants and fungi in the fight against infectious disease. A definitive guide for those who wish to study this in greater detail is *Herbal Medicine: Biomolecular and Clinical Aspects, Oxidative Stress and Disease*, second edition, edited by Iris FF Benzie and Sissi Wachtel-Galor.[54] Some work by killing microbes directly, but many of the beneficial effects result from impacts on the immune system. These can form an important part of improving the defences.

As an illustration of how clever these herbals can be, consider the life cycle of the beneficial fungus *Cordyceps*. Their fungal spores invade the larvae of insects and other 'creepy-crawlies'. Different species of *Cordyceps* are specific to, and invade, different larvae, including those of butterflies, moths, beetles, locusts, grasshoppers, spiders, cockroaches, ants, bees and probably others. The mycelia (the vegetative part of a fungus, consisting of a network of fine white filaments) enter the bloodstream and spread through the body of the caterpillar/larva, eventually killing it and mummifying the body but leaving the exoskeleton (outer casing) intact. The following summer it sprouts out through the head to form the mushroom. Consider, how do they recognise their particular host? How do they find the bloodstream of the larvae? How do they know which end is the head? If they can achieve so much, then killing microbes must be a 'piece of cake' by comparison!

Editor's note: Or as we used to say at my primary school, 'Easy peasy lemon squeezy'. Craig.

Historical note: The origin of this phrase is derived from an advertising slogan for the washing-up liquid Lemon Sqezy.

The starting point is to regularly consume any herb, spice or mushroom that you can get your hands on in large amounts. Initially at least, I do not think it matters much which you go for, because they all have antimicrobial benefits given they are all modern-day survivors. However, I am greatly influenced by taste, availability and, being naturally mean, cost. I am fortunate to have a garden with a variety of herbs which are a joy to collect and consume. Many do not even get into the kitchen – I am currently scoffing parsley, rocket and wild garlic. My good friend, Les, inoculated a stump with shitake and we now get mushrooms. I have made buckets of wood chips and piled them up in my polytunnel to grow oyster mushrooms. My favourite hill grows parasols and horse mushrooms in season. My top of the pops herbs for dishes I detail in *The PK Cookbook* include garlic, black pepper, ginger, rosemary, mint and thyme. I love Indian dishes with turmeric, cardamom, coriander and cumin. We are very fortunate to live in a world with access to all these delights.

Historical note: In AD 408, Attila the Hun demanded a huge quantity of pepper as ransom during the siege of Rome. One of the major reasons for Europe's expansion and eventual colonisation of southeast Asia was the pursuit of black pepper. In the 16th century, pepper was worth more than gold. It was so valuable that dock workers were prohibited from wearing clothing with pockets or cuffs for fear they would make off with the booty!

Much of the herbology that follows I have learned from the books of Stephen Buhner, medical herbalist. He has a similarly irreverent and refreshing view of orthodoxy. He likes to give his patients the knowledge and the tools of the trade so they can sort themselves out. In this respect, he is a disciple of Nicholas Culpepper, who likewise empowered his patients. Culpepper stated:

Three kinds of people mainly disease the people – priests, physicians and lawyers – priests disease matters belonging to their souls, physicians disease matters belonging to their bodies, and lawyers disease matters belonging to their estate.

Nicholas Culpepper, English botanist, herbalist, physician and author of *The English Physician* (1652) and *The Complete Herbal* (1653) (1616 – 1654)

Indeed, herbalism has a rich history stretching back much further than Culpeper. Sometime between AD 50 and 70, Pedanius Dioscorides, a Greek physician in the Roman army, wrote *De Materia Medica* (*On Medical Material*). This was a five-volume work covering many medicines and including about 600 plants and herbs, and listing 1000 medicines deriving from them. This tome lasted as the primary source of herbal medical knowledge for the next 1500 years. It is still in print today and runs to 913 pages.[55]

Back to the 21st century…Buhner has written several books, all a delight to read, with essential and useful practical clinical information.[8, 9]

Editorial note: I have very much enjoyed reading *Herbal Antibiotics* and *Herbal Antivirals* by Buhner, both of which arrived on my doorstep from a mystery benefactor – I suspect from one of the many wonderful members of the Dr Myhill Facebook group. Once you have followed the advice in this book, and also when you have become 'PK adapted', you will be able to enjoy his writing; your brain fog having lifted! – Craig

However, I suspect the abundance of information he supplies may make it difficult for the fatigued, foggy-brained, sick patient to know where to start. For details of the biology, pharmacology, cultivation, preparation, variety of uses and clinical applications you must read his books. Here I shall confine myself to the bare minimum of what you need to know to get started.

Remember, your best doctor will be yourself – the more you can understand the mechanisms of disease, the better able will you be at putting in place effective interventions. Our immune systems and defence mechanisms are as individual as our characters and personalities. Like the game of cricket, I can give you the general laws but you have to develop your own style within those rules. Boycott played a very different game from Botham, but both were highly effective at putting runs on the board.

Doctor: Therein the patient, Must minister to himself.

Macbeth: Throw physic to the door. I'll none of it.

Macbeth, Act 5, Scene 3, by William Shakespeare
(26 April 1564 (baptised) – 23 April 1616)

Buhner too recognises that there is a two-pronged approach to treating infection – first improve the defences, then kill the little wretches. Many herbs multitask, with properties in both departments. I have therefore picked out three herbs which improve the 'defences' (that is, support the immune system) and therefore have application in each and every infectious disease: namely *Astragalus*, *Cordyceps* and rhodiola. They have some additional antimicrobial actions as well as being immune-supportive. All three have the potential to help in fatigue syndromes because of a multiplicity of effects, improving mitochondrial function (and therefore immune function) and reducing any infectious load.

These herbs further qualify for inclusion because they are all extremely safe, remarkably free from side effects, delicious and relatively inexpensive. These are the real 'super foods'. *Astragalus* and *Cordyceps* should be included in one's regular diet as a food rather than as a medicine. Herbalism often overlaps with food history, in so far as many of the herbs historically used by humans to season food also protect against the threat of food-borne pathogens, either by supporting the immune system or by direct antimicrobial effect. The use of spices in India evolved partly to prevent meat rotting in the heat. Furthermore, like vitamin C and iodine, there is minimal potential for harm with self-medication using these herbs. All of them are considerably safer than sugar and fruit sugar. These three herbs would be an excellent starting point in the additional treatment (that is to say, over and above what has gone before in this book) with respect to the prevention and cure of acute and chronic infection.

Table 13.2: Herbs that can help us win the arms race

Herb	Effects	Dose	Notes
Astragalus (a legume)	Assists with delivery of energy and raw materials to foot soldiers and officers of the immune system Provides ammunition Improves communication to prevent friendly fire Helps to mop up the damage which inevitably results in killing zones Directly toxic to many viruses ('flu, HHV1, CMV, Hep B and others) Antibacterial (staph, strep, E coli, Lyme and others) Antifungal (candida)	Whole root powder 15-60 grams a day taken in three separate doses. Start with a low dose and build up. As with all antimicrobials in chronic infection, one can get a die off, or Herxheimer, reaction.* In this event reduce the dose a little, wait for the symptoms to settle and then retry a higher dose.	The sliced root in soup and stews is delicious It also makes a good tea – it has a slightly sweet taste It can be chewed raw as a chewing gum alternative
Cordyceps (a fungus)	Improves energy delivery from mitochondria Assists with delivery of energy and raw materials to foot soldiers and officers of the immune system Provides ammunition Improves communication to prevent friendly fire Helps to mop up the damage which inevitably results in killing zones Antiviral ('flu, HHV1, HIV, Hep B) Antibacterial (TB, staph, strep) Antifungal (candida) Kills *Mycoplasma*	Whole fungus 3-9 grams a day. Up to 50 grams a day in acute infection. May lower blood sugar so diabetics on medication must be aware – more reason to get PK-adapted (see page 234) before you start	The following makes a superb treat: Melt together equal weights of cocoa fat, coconut oil and *Cordyceps* powder. Tip some goji berries into paper cup cake moulds and cover with the melted mix. Store in, and eat directly from, the fridge

| Rhodiola (looks like a sedum) | Especially used for neuroprotection Improves energy delivery from mitochondria Assists with delivery of energy and raw materials to foot soldiers and officers of the immune system Provides ammunition Improves communication to prevent friendly fire Helps to mop up the damage which inevitably results in killing zones Antiviral ('flu, Hep C, coxsackie B) Antibacterial (staph, TB,) | Use the whole herb in capsules twice daily Up to 1000 milligrams daily Some people feel a bit jittery – I suspect this is due to low blood sugar. All the more reason to get PK-adapted | A teaspoon of leaves with boiling water poured over them makes a good tea |

*Table footnote: A Herxheimer reaction can be a reaction to endotoxin-like products released by the death of harmful microorganisms within the body. The contents of 'burst' microbial cells are released into the body and this has a temporary toxic effect until such toxins can be cleared out of the system; it can also be an allergy-like reaction (see page 232).

Let's leave the last word to Dioscorides, who, in his third volume, wrote this of *Astragalus*:

The roots (cut and smeared on) heal cut-apart sinews and wounds, and a decoction of it (taken as a drink) is good for disorders of the strength.[56]

Chapter 14

Use your brain

You were born with a perfectly good brain. Now is the time to use it!

Mrs Pearce, 1968, before every times-table test,
Princes Risborough County Middle School (Craig's first teacher)

The brain is just as important, and indeed as effective, as the immune system in disease prevention, but using our brain takes energy and we are naturally idle. Wake up and read on!

Avoid exposure to infection

Historically, the greatest reductions in infectious diseases have resulted from human intelligence, planning and organisation.

Historical note: Think of John Snow (15 March 1813 – 16 June 1858). In the 19th century, it was assumed that cholera was airborne. However, Snow did not accept this 'miasma' (bad air) theory. He argued that cholera in fact entered the body through the mouth. He published his ideas in an essay entitled *On the Mode of Communication of Cholera* in 1849. In August 1854, Snow proved his theory – a cholera outbreak occurred in Soho and after careful investigation, including plotting cases of cholera on a map of the area, Snow was able to identify a water

---

pump in Broad (now Broadwick) Street as the source of the disease. He had the handle of the pump removed and cases of cholera immediately began to diminish. Snow had used his brain to good effect and had reduced cases of cholera without the use of any drugs. Even so, his theory was not accepted until the 1860s.

But we don't all have to be John Snows – there are things we can do in our own lives that reduce our own individual chances of infection.

The obvious examples for us as individuals, as well as for society as a whole, include better nutrition and good hygiene, with clean water, air and food. With these interventions, Western killers such as cholera (*de quibus supra*), typhoid fever, tuberculosis, leprosy, plague, whooping cough, diphtheria, measles and other such diseases have greatly diminished. It is important to realise that these falls in disease impact pre-dated vaccination programmes (and the rate of decline did not change with vaccination). However, with the advent of antimicrobial drugs, we have been lulled into a false sense of security and we now have the expectation that as individuals we no longer need to use our brains. This has led to further risk-taking behaviours, some of which are an inevitable part of life… think the '4 Gs' – gobs, guts, genitals and gnats.

Table 14.1: The '4 Gs' routes of infection

Route of infection	At risk of	Leading to
Gobs	Glandular fever, 'mono' or Epstein Barr virus (EBV) – 'the kissing disease' – virus infects by saliva	CFS/ME, autoimmunity, cancer
Guts: Overseas travel – risk from unclean and microbiologically unfamiliar water and food	Gut parasites (*Giardia*, amoebiasis, *Blastocystis hominis*) Microbes different from those at home Enteroviruses	Traveller's diarrhoea Fermenting gut CFS/ME – I see many young people whose ME followed an overseas trip
Genitals	*Chlamydia*	Infertility CFS/ME

Route of infection	At risk of	Leading to
Genitals	HHV2 – genital herpes	Cancer – cervical; probably prostate
	HPV (human papilloma virus) – genital warts	Cancer
	Gonorrhoea	Infertility Increased risk of picking up other STDs
	Trichomoniasis	Ditto
		Post-viral chronic fatigue, autoimmunity and cancer
	Hepatitis B and C	Liver cirrhosis, cancer
	Retroviruses such as HIV	Death, dementia, cancer Immune suppression which increases the risk of acquiring and suffering all other infections
	Fungi such as candida	There is a clear link with endometriosis which, in turn, is a risk for cancer: ovarian, breast, brain and endocrine
	Syphilis – a classic example of an acute disease becoming chronic and killing	General paralysis of the insane Thankfully rare due to its effective treatment with penicillin
Gnats and other insect bites	Tropical diseases too numerous to list (malaria, Dengue etc) Lyme disease, *Bartonella* and *Babesia* are known to be spread by ticks but my guess is any biting insect may be a vector The Black Death, or plague, *Yersinia*, was spread by rat fleas *Rickettsia* (causes typhus)	Choose your holidays carefully! Avoid exposure Cover up and use mosquito netting Interventions to prevent disease can be equally damaging as evidenced by the drug Larium (used to prevent malaria) and pesticides to kill insects. Larium is now known to cause neurotoxicity.[57]

Intravenous drug abuse	HIV Hepatitis B Hepatitis C	As above. Avoid!
	Prion disorders	CJD and possibly other neurological diseases – Alzheimer's, Parkinson's and motor neurone disease are all prion disorders. (I have to say I would be nervous of having a blood transfusion)
Injuries: Cuts, wounds and burns	Skin is a vital defence Tetanus	Always consider the possibility of tetanus. This is the one vaccination I would recommend. If you are not vaccinated or not sure then go to hospital for an injection of tetanus antitoxin. Always clean any wound thoroughly, smother with iodine ointment 10%, cover and protect until the skin has healed over

We are incredibly fortunate to have some fantastic antimicrobial treatments for many of the above conditions. However, we cannot rely on these in the long term – microbes are cunning and antimicrobial resistance is constantly evolving. We should see these treatments as a window of opportunity to change our behaviour. Not to put ourselves at risk in the first place is always the best option.

An ounce of prevention is worth a pound of cure.

Benjamin Franklin (17 January 1706 – 17 April 1790)

Historical note: Franklin was one of the Founding Fathers of the United States of America but was something of a polymath – for example, he wrote an essay on *The Morals of Chess* (1786) in which he spoke of three key qualities: Foresight (consider the consequences of your actions), Circumspection (know the whole picture as well as you can) and Caution (never act too hastily). These qualities might serve us well when dealing with infections too.

Sex hormones

We have a particular problem with sex hormones, which put us at great risk of sexually transmitted disease (STDs). First, they induce a state of madness which makes us do crazy things. Secondly, they seem to wipe the memory so that these madnesses are repeated. I know this from my own experience. Whilst in labour with my firstborn, I told myself 'Never ever let yourself get into this ghastly situation ever again!' Within a year, I was again pregnant. My guess is that without this memory-deleting effect of sex hormones, women would never have more than one pregnancy and the species would disappear. Thankfully with age these madnesses decline somewhat…

Sex is an essential part of life and propagation of the species, but it bypasses our usual defences. Clever microbes have worked this out and made a living in this niche market.

The Pill

The contraceptive pill makes all the problems of STDs much worse for several reasons. Women can be sexually promiscuous without risk of pregnancy but at huge risk of STDs with multiple infections. Men have always been able to be sexually promiscuous without risk of pregnancy, but they are equally at huge risk of STDs with multiple infections. The Pill is immunosuppressive so infection is more likely. It is also growth-promoting so the cancer-generating effects of human papilloma virus (HPV) and human herpes virus (HHV1) are enhanced. We are seeing epidemics of infertility and cancer in young women and the Pill is greatly to blame.

Drugs that make things worse

We must also recognise that many drugs impair our defences against infection, as shown in Table 14.2.

Table 14.2: Drugs that impair our defences

Drug	Mechanism	Result
Acid-blocking drugs such as PPIs, H2 blockers, antacids – e.g. omeprazole, lansoprazole, ranitidine	Prevent the stomach concentrating acid	Microbes ingested or inhaled are not killed by stomach acid but go on to infect the rest of the gut and/or invade the bloodstream
	We need an acid stomach to digest protein and absorb minerals and vitamin B12	We deprive our standing army of essential raw materials
Diuretics	Increase the urinary excretion of essential minerals	We deprive our standing army of essential raw materials
Antibiotics	Damage the microbiome of the gut, mouth, vagina and bladder, especially if eating a high-carbohydrate diet	Fermenting gut by yeast Oral, vaginal and anal thrush Fermenting gut by unfriendly bacteria
Statins	Prevent the body from making its own coenyzme Q10	Mitochondria cannot work and so energy-delivery mechanisms are slowed; we cannot provide our standing army with energy
Beta blockers	Inhibit mitochondrial function	Ditto
Psychotropic drugs, e.g. antidepressants, tranquillisers	Many inhibit mitochondrial function	Ditto There is a difficult balance here – they may help sleep quantity, which is an essential part of energy-delivery mechanisms, but they may also worsen sleep quality
Steroids, NSAIDs, paracetamol, cancer chemotherapy	Suppress the immune system	Prevents our standing army from responding (However, these drugs may be helpful if the standing army is in inappropriate overdrive)
Asthma inhalers Steroid sprays and skin creams	Suppress the immune system Open up the bronchi and allow pathogens in	Ditto above

Drug	Mechanism	Result
Morphine, codeine and other such powerful painkillers	Suppress the immune system	Ditto The progress of cancer is accelerated once morphine drugs are prescribed[58, 58a]
Recognise that many cough-and-cold remedies …	…are symptom suppressing…	…with the potential to do harm – they impair our defences and prevent our immune system from doing its job
Antipsychotic drugs	Raise blood sugar, induce metabolic syndrome and possibly lead to diabetes	Increase the risk of all infections
Sunscreens	Block ultraviolet light and prevent vitamin D synthesis in the skin	Vitamin D deficiency increases the risk of all infections

The trouble with vaccinations

We also need to recognise that vaccination is not as effective as we might want to believe.

We live in times of news and fake news. Big Pharma has relied on fake news for decades and nowhere more so than in the field of vaccination. This has been unravelled and detailed by investigative journalist Christina England and scientist Lucija Tomljenovic, PhD, in their magnificent book *Vaccination Policy and the UK Government: The Untold Truth*.[59] It has been gorgeously researched and referenced, contains extensive and astonishing quotes and makes for gripping reading. It has given me several sleepless nights. With their permission, I am repeating the chapter summaries below with some of my straight-talking additions. All potential vaccine recipients, and parents of vaccine recipients, should read this book before accepting any vaccination.

Indeed, I have seen so many children with autism, convulsions and CFS/ME following vaccination that I have no doubt of the veracity of this book. Autism is the most expensive Western disease, now afflicting 1 in 64 of children in the UK.[60, 61] Here is a brief summary of their findings, with any direct quotes in italics.

Table 14.3: Summary of *Vaccination Policy and the UK Government: The Untold Truth*

Chapters and sections	Main issue	Selected quote from
Part 1: Introduction by Dr Michael Innis, Haematologist	Medical policy is determined by Big Pharma with profits in mind. Potential benefits and side-effects are secondary issues.	*The authors have provided a treasury of facts and figures exposing all that is undesirable in the current medico-pharmacological environment (page 10)*
1. Vaccination and corruption in Government	Members of the following committees all had extensive links to Big Pharma: • Committee on Safety of Medicines 1989 • Sub-committee on adverse reactions to vaccines and immunological products 1989 • Sub-committee on adverse reactions to vaccines and immunisations 1990 advising on vaccine safety and effectiveness • Sub-committee on adverse reactions to vaccines and immunisation 1991	*Professor Sir Roy Meadow, who was a member of all these committees, was a share-holder in Boots and Beecham and declared that his department received fees from the pharmaceutical industry (pages 23-26)*
2. Joining the dots – Shoot the whistle blower	Clinical psychologist Lisa Blakemore Brown demonstrated how doctors were ignoring post-vaccination events, such as cot death and autism. Instead, parents were blamed for their child's illness. She was vilified by her peers and her career was sabotaged.	
3. Lifting the lid off Pandora's box	Gulf War syndrome (GWS) is clearly linked to multiple vaccinations. (It is my clinical experience that many cases of GWS were triggered by vaccination. I saw one patient who received 14 vaccinations on one day in Germany and these were all repeated one month later in the Gulf. His medical records were destroyed by the MoD.)	*Soldiers received the following vaccinations: yellow fever, typhoid, cholera, hepatitis A, hepatitis B, meningitis, anthrax, pertussis and plague (pages 88-89)* *They also received a dangerous MMR vaccine called Pluserix. This had already been withdrawn from use in Canada because of high levels of adverse reactions in children (page 93)*

Chapters and sections	Main issue	Selected quote from
4. The case of Christina England	She was falsely accused of Munchausen's syndrome by proxy when one of her adopted sons suffered adverse reactions following an MMR vaccination	Blame the patient or, even better, the patient's mother
Part 2: Introduction	Vaccination policy and the UK government: a total lack of transparency	*British health authorities have been deliberately concealing information from parents for the sole purpose of getting them to comply with an "official" vaccination schedule.* (page 141)
5. How the Joint Committee on Vaccination and Immunisation (JCVI) fudged and covered up report of adverse effects	*The UK health authorities continued to promote the MMR vaccine as safe despite the fact that the Urabe strain mumps component of the vaccine was unambiguously demonstrated by their own investigations to trigger aseptic meningitis in certain children* (page 144)	*The Department of Health was compelled to action only when the vaccine manufacturer, on the advice of their lawyers, decided to stop producing the vaccine.* (page 144)
6. Ditto above	*The JCVI restricted the contraindications to pertussis vaccination in order to boost vaccination rates in spite of unsettling safety data and uncertainties concerning the actual risk/benefit balance of pertussis vaccination in vulnerable children who were potentially more at risk of vaccine-associated adverse outcomes* (p158)	*...by persistently restricting vaccination contraindication criteria so more children could be vaccinated...the JCVI appeared to have prioritised vaccination policy over vaccine safety.* (page 158)
7. JCVI are more worried about profit than people	*The UK health authorities sought to conceal their documented conclusions on the possible link between DPT [diphtheria, pertussis (whooping cough) and tetanus] vaccination and serious neurological illness due to concerns of legal repercussions* (page 165)	*The JCVI furthermore, on multiple occasions, requested from vaccine manufacturers to make specific amendments to their data sheets, when these were in conflict with the JCVI's official advices on immunisations* (page 165)

8. The JCVI cherry-picked the data to suit their desired outcome	*The JCVI persistently relied on methodologically dubious studies, while dismissing independent research, in order to promote vaccine policies* (page 173)	*Cochrane 2005 MMR review "The design and reporting of safety outcomes in MMR vaccine studies, both pre and post marketing, are largely inadequate"* (page 173)
9. Money beats Truth	The JCVI persistently and categorically downplayed safety concerns while over-inflating vaccine benefits	*Since the introduction of mumps vaccination in 1967 peak incidence has moved from 5-9 years to 10-24 years. Serious complications have risen as a consequence with mumps orchitis... [which] leads to male sterility* (page 184)
10. Ditto	*The JCVI promoted and elaborated a plan for introducing the new unlicensed meningococcal C conjugate vaccines into the routine paediatric schedule based on limited safety data and, by their own admission, lack of good evidence for the vaccines' efficacy, on the assumption that the licenses would eventually be granted* (page 191)	
11. Don't look and you won't see	*The UK authorities actively discouraged further research on vaccine associated sudden infant death syndrome claiming that such research would give allegedly undue credibility to vaccine safety concerns* (page 198)	
12. The mushroom education: keep 'em in the dark and feed them bullshit	*The UK health authorities took advantage of parents' trust and lack of relevant knowledge on vaccinations in order to promote a poorly tested immunisation schedule* (page 202)	*...the vaccine was demonstrated safe based on a seven-day follow-up and monitoring for largely local reactions. Seven days is a totally inadequate follow-up time* (page 203)

Vaccination causes much more disease than it prevents. The infectious diseases involved can be easily, safely and effectively prevented and treated with all the tools of the trade detailed in this book. Most do not need professional help. You can do it yourself! Do Groundhog Basic (page 98), stock up your first aid box (see page 215), use your brain and you will be ready for anything.

Do not ignore symptoms and do not suppress symptoms with drugs!

When we get sick we develop symptoms and they are a vital part of our defences. Symptom-suppressing drugs should not be used because they increase the numbers of invaders and decrease our defences for the obvious reasons detailed in Table 14.4.

Table 14.4: The benefits of the symptoms of infection

Symptom	Mechanism	Do not symptom suppress
Fatigue	Makes us rest so that the immune system has the necessary energy to fight	Caffeine and pseudoephedrine give us false energy
Fever	Most microbes are heat sensitive – a good fever kills them directly	Aspirin, NSAIDs and paracetamol prevent us running a temperature. Wrap up and keep warm. Sweat it out!
Malaise and prostration Muscle aches and joint pains	Makes you keep still. This allows our soldiers to fight on *terra firma* This also saves physical energy	Do not use NSAIDs and paracetamol. Lie still instead. Rest.
Lots of mucus in the nose and throat	Provides a sticky surface to trap microbes (this was a major reason why Henry V beat the French at Agincourt in 1415 – the French armoured knights wallowed into the mud and could not fight effectively)	Pseudoephedrine dries up mucus production and allows microbes to get into the body
Cough, sneeze and spit	Physically expels microbes from the body (Of course, this also helps to spread microbes – I told you they were clever little sods. Some people are not bright enough to reduce this spread with a handkerchief)	Codeine suppresses coughs. Hawking up sputum and spitting in public was made socially unacceptable, helping reduce the spread of TB

Runny nose	Ditto	Pseudoephedrine dries up mucus production. However, this is short lived – if used regularly one gets 'rebound hypersecretion' as the body compensates – well done the body!
Bronchospasm and wheeze	Narrowing the airways greatly increases the turbulence of air flowing through the passages so microbes get flung out and stuck on the mucous lining.	Inhalers open up the airways – they must be use judiciously; they may allow microbes to penetrate deeper into the lungs
Loss of appetite, nausea	Keep the stomach empty so that the microbes stuck onto mucus are coughed up and end in an acid bath that has not been diluted by food	If you do not feel like eating then do not! Do not snack Take vitamin C to bowel tolerance (see page 57)
	Sugar and carbs feed microbes. The immune system prefers to run on fat. Even a lean athlete has the necessary fat stores to feed the immune system for days	Do not eat sugar and carbs. Remember, fruit is a bag of sugar
Feel and look miserable. Children and men grizzle and moan – we are back to 'man 'flu'!	This induces an empathetic response in fellow humans. Women generally are better at this than men. They swing into action. with warm blankets and hot water bottles. They administer the vitamins and herbals detailed in this book, take on all the jobs that the patient normally does and make jolly, cooing noises like 'never mind, darling, you'll be fine in a day or two'	It is my experience that men are much better at looking miserable than women. (Sorry Craig. Well done, Penny) (Guilty as charged, M'ladies. Craig)

In short, our symptoms are 'meant' to make us behave in certain ways, which will help us to fight off the infection. To suppress these symptoms is to suppress the evolutionary 'memory' of our immune systems. And these combined 'memories' of our immune system inform our bodies how to act and behave during an infection.

It's a poor sort of memory that only works backwards!

Lewis Carroll (1832 – 1898), *Alice in Wonderland*

Be positive

All the functions of the brain are reflected in the immune system, which I see as a mobile brain. We know that having an optimistic, sunny disposition is good for immunity. I imagine people with such characters have jolly white cells like the knights of King Arthur who rush around on white chargers killing off the baddies. So much of modern medicine is disempowering. I find simply explaining to my patients what is going wrong, why it is going wrong and how they can fight disease instantly supplies the very positive mental attitude they need to recover.

Take control. Just do it!

Personal note from Craig: This was certainly true in my case. With the notable exception of Sarah, all my previous doctors and health professionals had made their best attempts to 'ignore' what was going on inside my body and all had encouraged me to do likewise. I was told not to read books or search the internet because this would confuse and upset me. Well, nothing could be further from the truth – the moment I began to understand what was going wrong inside my body, my entire outlook changed in a blink of an eye. Once I had done this research I understood my illness, and this knowledge was based on fact, rather than on the intellectually risible and totally un-evidenced conjectures about my illness that I had been told by the established medical profession for years. Now I had an enemy in my sights and I could do something about it!

Summary

Remember to use your brain to:
- Avoid infections where you can – Franklin's 'Foresight'
- Be aware that some drugs impair your ability to fight infections – Franklin's 'Circumspection'
- Understand that vaccinations are not all they might seem – Franklin's 'Caution'.

Chapter 15

Groundhog Basic

Because I constantly refer back to this basic approach which is fundamental to the treatment of all infections, from here on I will call this 'Groundhog Basic' or simply 'Groundhog'. In the film *Groundhog Day*, the main protagonist finds himself in an ever-recurring time loop that gives him the opportunity to put things right; Groundhog Basic is another sort of loop that also bears constant repetition. The point here is that Groundhog done well and in a timely manner will prevent acute illness developing and chronic disease getting a foothold.

It is also the case that Groundhog will need to change through life as we are exposed to new infections and as our defences decline with age. All of us should do the **Groundhog Basic** all (well, most) of the time. All should be prepared to upgrade to **Groundhog Acute** (page 110) to deal with unexpected and sudden infectious challenges (get that First Aid box stocked up now – see Appendix 1). All will need to move to **Groundhog Chronic** (page 174) as we age and acquire an infectious load.

It is so important to have all the following in place and then at the first sign of any infection take vitamin C to bowel tolerance (that is, an amount that causes diarrhoea – see page 57) and use iodine for local infections because:

1. You will feel much better very quickly!
2. The immune system will not be so activated that it cannot turn off subsequently. So many patients I see with ME started their illness with an acute infection from which they never recovered – the immune system stayed switched on.

Groundhog Basic

Table 15.1: How to do Groundhog Basic

The paleo-ketogenic (PK) diet: High fat, high fibre, very low carb Probiotic foods like kefir and sauerkraut No dairy or grains Two meals a day; no snacking	See our books *Prevent and Cure Diabetes – delicious diets not dangerous drugs* for the 'why' and *The PK Cookbook – go paleo-ketogenic and get the best of both worlds* for the 'how'.
A basic package of nutritional supplements – multi-vitamins, multi-minerals and vitamin D	A good multivitamin and sunshine salt (1 teaspoon daily with food). A dessertspoon of hemp oil.
Vitamin C	Take vitamin C (5 grams) last thing at night; this stays in the gut undiluted by food for best effect.
Sleep 8-9 hours between 10:00 pm and 7:00 am	More in winter, less in summer.
Exercise at least once a week when you push yourself to your limit	It is anaerobic exercise that produces lactic acid and stimulates new muscle fibres and new mitochondria to develop.
Herbs, spices and fungi in cooking	Use your favourite herbs, spices and fungi in cooking and food, and lots of them – yum yum!
If fatigue is an issue, address energy delivery mechanisms as best you can	See our book *Diagnosis and Treatment of Chronic Fatigue Syndrome and Myalgic Encephalitis: it's mitochondria, not hypochondria.*
Heat and light	Keep warm. Sunbathe at every opportunity.
Use your brain	Foresight: Avoid risky actions like kissing* and unprotected sex. Caution: Avoid vaccinations. Travel with care. Circumspection: Do not suppress symptoms with drugs; treat breaches of the skin seriously. See Chapter 7, page 43.

*Table footnote: Oscar Wilde (16 October 1854 – 30 November 1900) knew this, perhaps for different reasons than the risk of infection, when he wrote that: 'A kiss may ruin a human life' (from *A Woman of No Importance*. (Is there ever such a thing? Craig)

3. The shorter and less severe the acute infection, the less chance of switching

on inappropriate immune reactions, such as autoimmunity. Many viruses are associated with an arthritis – so-called 'palindromic rheumatism'. I think of this as viral allergy.

4. The shorter and less severe the acute infection, the less chance the microbe has of making itself a permanent home in your body. As you have read (Chapter 2), many diseases – from Crohn's and cancer to polymyalgia and Parkinson's – have an infectious driver.

Note: Palindromic rheumatism is rheumatism that comes and goes. The word 'palindrome' was coined by English playwright Ben Johnson in the 17th Century from the Greek roots *palin* (πάλιν; 'again') and *dromos* (δρόμος; 'way', 'direction'). The first known palindrome, written as a graffito, and etched into the walls of a house in Herculaneum, reads thus:

sator arepo tenet opera rotas – 'The sower Arepo leads with his hand the plough.' [idiomatic translation]

Many of the graffiti (graffito is the singular of graffiti) found in Pompeii and Herculaneum are somewhat bawdy, some focusing on what the local ladies of the fine houses would like to do with certain named gladiators or, indeed, vice versa… the authors leave it to the readers to do their own research.

So, are you back with us yet? We will now look further at the enemy.

Part III

How to treat acute infections that have got past our defences

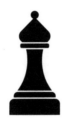

Chapter 16

Who is the enemy?

Usually the enemy is our neighbour, living right inside us. As GK Chesterton (English writer, poet, philosopher, dramatist, journalist, orator, lay theologian, biographer, and literary and art critic (1874 – 1935)) said:

The Bible tells us to love our neighbours, and also to love our enemies; probably because generally they are the same people.

Well, we shall ignore this Biblical advice to love our enemies… but we should certainly get to know them. There are literally millions of microbes and parasites aching to make themselves at home in our comfortable bodies. However, for the practical purposes of this book it's useful to think of them in the following three groups: (1) microbes that we have lived with amicably for millions of years; (2) traditional, or well known, enemy microbes; and (3) 'emerging microbes'.

1. Symbiotic microbes

These are microbes that have been with us for millions of years and made themselves at home in the human body. In fact, we have harnessed them to help us so they are not parasites but 'symbiotes'. The body has learned how to deal with them and keep them at bay. In all cases, maintain the body's defences with Groundhog Basic with special attention to the items in Table 16.1.

Table 16.1: Symbiotic microbes and how to live comfortably with them

Examples	How to deal with them / how they infect us / resulting problems etc
Gut microbiome – the collection of micro-organisms living within the gut. These microbes do lots of useful jobs such as: • fermenting fibre to become a useful fuel – namely, short chain fatty acids • physically crowding out invaders, thereby protecting us from infection • making some useful molecules, such as vitamin K2, serotonin • training and programming our immune system in the gut.	The PK diet (see page 234).
Skin and mucous membrane flora	Do not kill these with antibiotic soaps or aluminium-based deodorants. Indeed, do not wash too much or you will wash off the friendly skin flora. In my family it used to be a weekly bath… and we shared the same bath water!
Human virome – the collection of viruses in and on the human body, such as bacteriophages, which make up 15% of the gut microbiome. Some viruses are integrated into the genome. Viruses can be found on all skin and mucous surfaces.	We are stuck with these – but we all carry a similar load, so the playing field is flat. Do not risk adding to this load with vaccinations.

2. Traditional enemy microbes

These are microbes that have been our enemies for years but through our intelligence and organisation we have learned to deal with.

• In all cases, prevent by maintaining the defences with Groundhog Basic.
• Attack any infection at the first sign with Groundhog Acute – see Chapter 17, page 110.

Table 16.2: Traditional enemy microbes and how to deal with them

Microbe/condition	Notes – how to deal with them
Cholera	Clean water to drink
Polio	Clean water to bathe in
Other enteroviruses – picorna, Coxsackie A and B, ECHO virus E 71	Spread by direct contact and water (survive freezing and chlorination). These are a major trigger for CFS/ME. Cause epidemics of gastroenteritis. Coxsackie causes meningitis, carditis.
Tuberculosis Anthrax Influenza Whooping cough Pneumonia and chest infections Ebola and Marburg	Clean air (free from cigarette smoke, pollution and infection). Early diagnosis and isolation of acute cases. PK diet and nutritional supplements are highly protective.
Puerperal fever	Hand washing and excellent basic hygiene.
Anthrax Tetanus	Handwashing after handling infected livestock – e.g. goats, cattle, sheep. Spores are present in the soil so observe excellent basic hygiene
Hepatitis A *Salmonella* *Yersinia* Infectious gastroenteritis 'Worms' Gut parasites	Clean food to eat Good stomach acid from good PK diet
Meningitis – bacterial Epstein Barr virus	Kissing can spread infection – that is, avoid kissing an infected person!
Meningitis – viral	Faeces (e.g. when changing a nappy) can carry infection.
Hepatitis B, hepatitis C, HIV, syphilis, *Chlamydia* Jakob Creutzfeldt disease HTVL1 Zika virus	Practise safe sex. Use clean blood products and clean needles.

Microbe/condition	Notes – how to deal with them
HPV (human papilloma virus)	Practise safe sex
Malaria Bubonic plague Ebola and Marburg Dengue fever Yellow fever Zika virus	Keep free of insect bites
Rabies	Keep free of biting dogs and bats
Middle East respiratory syndrome	Keep free of fruit-eating bats
Hantavirus	Keep free of rats.

3. Emerging microbes

These are the new, unfamiliar enemy microbes that are emerging as a result of Western lifestyles (eroding the immune system) and climate change. We are acquiring these because of poor immune system defences. As these microbes may get in 'under the radar' we can call them 'stealth infections' (see Chapter 28). Having got into the body they create their own defences, part of which involves biofilm (page 191) and part disabling our immune system in cunning ways.

If the infection has become established and is driving a disease pathology, then we need to use Groundhog Chronic (page 174), almost certainly with additional antimicrobials in large doses, often in combination and for long duration.

Table 16.3: Newly emerging infections and their consequences

Chronic infection with 'X' and so driving …	…early, mid and late pathology…
MRSA and other antibiotic-resistant bacteria, such as SARS	They get into the body through direct contamination of open wounds: • **Early:** infected lesions that do not heal with antibiotics • **Mid:** infection spreads to other areas such as bone • **Late:** septicaemia and death.
Lyme disease (*Borrelia*)	Via tick bites, indeed, probably any insect bites; those with poor immune system defences risk systemic infection: • **Immediate:** rash and arthritis • **Mid:** myalgic encephalitis (ME) • **Late:** neurodegenerative disease such as dementia.
Chlamydia	Ditto above.
Bartonella, Babesia	Ditto above.
Yersinia	Acquired from contaminated food: • **Early:** enterocolitis • **Mid:** myalgic encephalitis (ME), tuberculosis-like disease.
Herpes virus 1 (HHV1)	Acquired through direct contact: • **Early:** local cold sore • **Late:** myasthenia gravis, melanoma, dementia.
HHV2 (genital herpes)	Acquired by direct contact: • **Early:** warts • **Late:** cervical cancer, cancer of penis, anus and vagina
HHV3 – chickenpox and shingles	Acquired through infection from others who have either acute chickenpox or acute shingles. Shingles cannot be 'caught'; it has to be already present in the body following a previous attack of chickenpox. If the immune system weakens the virus will wake up to cause shingles. • **Early:** blistering lesions • **Late:** leukaemia, lymphoma, breast cancer

Chronic infection with 'X' and so driving ...	...early, mid and late pathology...
HHV4 EBV (Epstein Barr virus) – this is a really nasty virus	Saliva, kissing • **Early:** glandular fever • **Mid:** ME (epidemics of!), 33 autoimmune conditions including systemic lupus erythematosus (SLE), multiple sclerosis (MS), rheumatoid arthritis, Sjorgren's • **Late:** Burkitt's lymphoma, nasopharyngeal cancer, stomach cancer, Hodgkin's disease
HHV5 (cytomegalovirus)	From body fluids (e.g. urine, saliva, blood, tears) • **Early:** glandular fever-like illness • **Mid:** ME • **Late:** prostate cancer, brain tumours (glioblastoma), Guillain Barre syndrome
HHV6 (roseola)	Respiratory fluids and saliva (coughing, sneezing, kissing) • **Early:** 'flu-like symptoms with rash and swollen lymph nodes • **Mid:** ME, Hashimoto's thyroiditis, temporal lobe epilepsy • **Late:** MS, lymphoma, leukaemia, brain tumours, Alzheimer's disease
HHV7 (roseola-like)	Acquired by many in early childhood but only manifests with immunosuppression • **Early:** 'flu-like symptoms with rash and swollen lymph nodes • **Mid:** ME, Grave's disease • **Late:** Alzheimer's disease
HIV	Sexual intercourse, blood transfusion, sharing needles • **Early:** 'flu-like symptoms • **Mid:** progressive immune suppression to the clinical picture of AIDS • **Late:** susceptibility to infections, dementia. HIV plus HHV7 may progress to Kaposi's sarcoma, lymphoma.
XMRV	Acquired through vaccination: • ME • prostate cancer.

Now that we know our new, emerging stealth diseases, let us learn how to beat them in the arms race. Our greatest weapons are Groundhog Basic, Groundhog Acute and Groundhog Chronic, and we can all do it!

I am quite sure that by now any intelligent reader will have adopted the principles of Groundhog Basic but what to do if that fails and you pick up an acute infection? Well, then you move to Groundhog Acute. Read on!

Figure 16.1: Explaining the Groundhogs

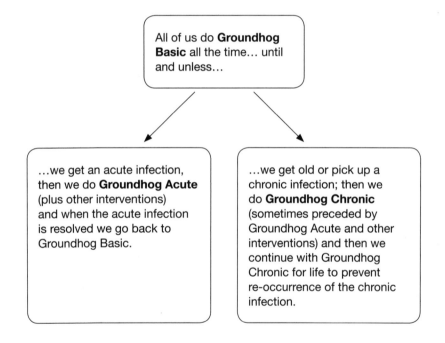

All of us do **Groundhog Basic** all the time… until and unless…

…we get an acute infection, then we do **Groundhog Acute** (plus other interventions) and when the acute infection is resolved we go back to Groundhog Basic.

…we get old or pick up a chronic infection; then we do **Groundhog Chronic** (sometimes preceded by Groundhog Acute and other interventions) and then we continue with Groundhog Chronic for life to prevent re-occurrence of the chronic infection.

Chapter 17

Groundhog Acute

At the first sign of any infection you must immediately put in place Groundhog Acute. Do not forget Dr Fred Klenner's advice:

The patient should get large doses of vitamin C in all pathological conditions while the physician ponders the diagnosis.

Dr Frederick Robert Klenner BS MS MD FCCP FAAFP (1907 – 1984)

Strike soon and strike hard because time is of the essence. It is worth repeating myself as the following is so important:

1. You will feel much better very quickly!
2. The immune system will not be so activated that it cannot turn off subsequently. So many patients I see with ME started their illness with an acute infection from which they never recovered – the immune system stayed switched on.
3. The shorter and less severe the acute infection, the less chance of switching on inappropriate immune reactions such as autoimmunity. Many viruses are associated with an arthritis – so-called 'palindromic rheumatism' (see page 100). I think of this as viral allergy.
4. The shorter and less severe the acute infection, the less the chance the microbe has of making itself a permanent home in your body. As you have read, many diseases from Crohn's and cancer, polymyalgia and Parkinson's to ME and malignancy all have an infectious driver.

At the first sign of the tingling, sore throat, runny nose, malaise, headache, cystitis, skin inflammation, insect bite, or whatever, follow the instructions in Table 17.1.

Table 17.1: What to do at the first sign of an infection

What to do	Why and how
The paleo-ketogenic diet: * high fat, high fibre, very low carb * probiotic foods like kefir and sauerkraut * no dairy or grains. Just two meals a day and no snacking.	See our books *Prevent and Cure Diabetes – delicious diets not dangerous drugs* for the 'why' and *The PK Cookbook – go paleo-ketogenic and get the best of both worlds* for the 'how'
You may consider a fast – this is essential for any acute gut infection. Drink rehydrating fluids – i.e. Sunshine salt (5 grams in 1 litre of water) *ad lib*	'Starve a cold; starve a fever' (No – not a typo – starve any short-lived infection)
Vitamin C to bowel tolerance. The need for vitamin C increases hugely with any infection. Interestingly, the bowel tolerance (the amount that induces diarrhoea) changes so one needs a much higher dose to get a loose bowel motion during an infection. If you do not have a very loose bowel motion within one hour, take another 10 grams. Keep repeating until you get diarrhoea Most need 3-4 doses to abolish symptoms	Vitamin C greatly reduces any viral, indeed any microbial, load in the gut. (Remember, some of the infecting load of influenza virus will get stuck onto the sticky mucus which lines the lungs and is coughed up and swallowed) Vitamin C improves the acid bath of the stomach Vitamin C protects us from the inevitable free-radical damage of an active immune system
A good multivitamin Sunshine salt (5 grams/1 teaspoon daily in water) A dessertspoon of hemp oil	Sunshine salt in water because you should be fasting – 5 grams (one teaspoonful) in one litre of water provides a 0.5% solution
Take Lugol's iodine 12% 2 drops in a small glass of water every hour until symptoms resolve; swill this round your mouth, gargle, sniff and inhale the vapour	30 seconds of direct contact with iodine kills all microbes
With respiratory symptoms, put 4 drops of Lugol's iodine 12% into a salt pipe and inhale for two minutes – do this at least four times a day Apply a smear of iodine ointment inside the nostrils	30 seconds of direct contact with iodine kills all microbes; iodine ointment in the nostrils will contact-kill microbes on their way in or on their way out, rendering you less infectious to others! (Remember to breathe through your nose, not your mouth)

What to do	Why and how
Apply iodine ointment 10% to any bite, skin break or swelling	Iodine ointment contact-kills all microbes and is absorbed through the skin to kill invaders
Herbs, spices and fungi	If you are still struggling, then go to Chapter 13 for the effective herbal preparations
Rest – listen to your symptoms and abide by them. Sleep is even more important with illness. Hippocrates said 'Give me a medicine to produce a fever, and I can cure any disease.' We don't need a medicine – the body gives us the fever that Hippocrates wanted. See below	I see so many people who push on through acute illness and risk a slow resolution of their disease with all the complications that accompany such. The immune system needs the energy to fight. I find vitamin C to bowel tolerance combined with a good night's sleep has kept me cold free and 'flu free for 35 years
Heat – keep warm	Fevers kill all microbes; you can get some benefit from sauna-ing. Do not exercise as you need the energy for your immune system
Light – sunshine is best	Sunbathe if possible
Use your brain – do not suppress symptoms with drugs	Symptoms help the body fight infection. Anti-inflammatories inhibit healing and repair – they allow the microbes to make themselves permanently at home in the body
If you develop other acute symptoms, read on…	…turn to the relevant chapters that follow, which all start with Groundhog Acute.

You may consider that doing all the above amounts to over-kill, but when that 'flu epidemic arrives, as it surely will, you will be very happy to have been prepared and to have these weapons to hand so that you, your family, friends and neighbours will survive. Stock up that first aid box now (see page 215).

'Be prepared'

Lord Baden-Powell in *Scouting for Boys*

and let us end with more wisdom from Benjamin Franklin (17 January 1706 – 17 April 1790):

By failing to prepare, you are preparing to fail.

Chapter 18

Acute coughs, colds, 'flus and their complications

What to do when you know you are becoming ill but do not yet know why

...no time like the present...

Old English proverb

Historical note: This proverb can be traced back to 1562, in Legh's *Accidence of Armoury*. Gerard Legh (died 1563) was a lawyer and this was his only work, and concerned the theories of gentility and living a heraldic life. Source: *Dictionary of Proverbs* (Wordsworth Reference) by George Latimer Apperson.

If you find yourself turning straight to this chapter because you are getting a cold or becoming 'flu-ey, do not waste time with anything else but go straight for vitamin C and iodine in proper doses, as explained in Groundhog Acute (page 110). Make a mental note that once you have recovered you should continue with Groundhog Basic (page 98) for life.

Translating the immunology into what you actually do

So how do all the previous chapters translate into what you actually do at the first sign of any illness, such as a cough and cold, which may or may not progress to a nasty 'flu, gut infection, urinary tract infection, chest infection or whatever? In the early stages neither you nor your doctor can know what the actual diagnosis is so we recommend the interventions in Table 18.1, which expand on Groundhog Acute.

You may discover a few critical interventions that do it for you; everyone is different.

Including the 'why' in Table 18.1, and in the previous chapters, should help to give the intellectual imperative to do the action; the 'why' is the 'translation', and although Cervantes (1547 – 1616, author of *Don Quixote*) said that 'translation is like looking at the other side of the tapestry' in a derogatory way, implying that the translated version was imperfect or not beautiful, I take the opposite view – by looking at the stitches, one can determine the mechanism of such stitching and then one can do something about it!

Table 18.1: What to do when there are signs of an unknown infection

Clinical symptoms and signs	What to do?	Why?
At the first sign of the tingling, sore throat, runny nose, malaise etc which means you are going to get something… which may be a common cold…	Take vitamin C to bowel tolerance (page 57). The need for vitamin C increases hugely with any infection. Interestingly, one's bowel tolerance changes so one needs a much higher dose to get a loose bowel motion during an infection. (I reckon I need 10 grams over and above my normal daily consumption to get a result.) If you do not have a very loose bowel motion within one hour, take another 10 grams. Keep repeating until you get diarrhoea. Remember: 'The patient should get large doses of vitamin C in all pathological conditions while the physician ponders the diagnosis.' Dr Fred R Klenner (22 October 1907 – 20 May 1984)	Vitamin C greatly reduces any viral, indeed any microbial, load in the gut. (Remember, some of the infecting load of any air-borne virus (e.g. influenza virus) will get stuck onto the sticky mucus which lines the lungs and is coughed up and swallowed.) Vitamin C: • improves the acid bath of the stomach • protects one from the inevitable free-radical damage of an active immune system • has worked brilliantly for me for years – but as I get older and the defences decline I may need some more ammo…
	Use iodine ointment 10% or Lugol's iodine 12% topically as described in Chapter 10 (page 61)	Remember, 30 seconds of contact kills all microbes

	With respiratory symptoms put 4 drops of Lugol's iodine 12% into a salt pipe and inhale for two minutes – do this at least four times a day	Ditto
	Apply a smear of iodine ointment 10% inside the nostrils	This will contact-kill microbes on their way in or out, rendering you less infectious to others
	Take *Bee Prepared* which is an excellent all-rounder – the bees got there before Baden-Powell (see Chapter 17 and page 218)	Bees protect their honey stores with bees' wax, propolis and other such – this has broad antimicrobial properties
	Take zinc and vitamin C lozenges every hour	Both zinc and vitamin C kill viruses directly but they must come into direct contact with the virus, ideally before it gets into the body
	Take selenium – chew a 100-mcgm capsule of selenium in the mouth up to five times daily	Again, direct contact with the virus is needed to be effective
	Take echinacea. Use tincture of *Echinacea angustiflora* – a few drops dribbled into your mouth as often as you can. Hold this in your mouth for as long as you can, gargle with it, and let it dribble slowly down your throat. I have one patient who stands on his head to allow it to soak the top of his throat and nasal passages… why not?	Again, direct contact with the virus is needed to be effective. **Note from Craig:** I used to buy my sweets from a shop called Tiffany's named after the proprietor. He was a great believer in the health benefits of standing on his head. Many was the time I went into his shop for my quarter of 'Rhubarb and Custard' only to be greeted by a pair of feet sticking in the air behind the counter. I would place my order, get the sweets myself and leave my 6d on the counter. Of course, this was pre PK diet

Clinical symptoms and signs	What to do?	Why?
	Elderberry syrup 800 mg/teaspoon – one teaspoon every waking hour Berberine (goldenseal) 800 mg chewed three times daily	This does not taste great, but hey ho…. Perhaps the Chinese proverb 'Good medicine for health tastes bitter to the mouth' has some truth in it?
	Rest and keep warm	See Groundhog Acute (page 110)
	Do not suppress symptoms with drugs	See Groundhog Acute
	Remember, ideally you should fast but certainly, no dairy products	Dairy products worsen catarrhal symptoms
	No carbs, especially no fruit, no sugar and no honey	These all feed microbes directly
If you may be progressing to influenza…	Increase the following from Groundhog Basic: • *Astragalus* to 50 grams • *Cordyceps* to 9 grams • rhodiola to 1 gram Add Chinese skullcap 1 gram every hour Liquorice 750 mg every hour *Lomatium* (Lomatin)	See Chapter 4 for how clever microbes are, with 'flu as a prime example

All the above interventions are effective for viral, bacterial and fungal infections. However, if the body's immune system has been compromised (which may be by scar tissue, the presence of established chronic infection (such as HIV or Lyme), poor immune function or poor energy delivery mechanisms), then you may well need other medical interventions. However, whatever you need, continue with all the above. The more ways one can fight infection, the better the success rate. My experience is that if all the above interventions are in place, then for someone who would otherwise be fairly fit and well, the need for further measures is rare. Should you need antibiotics, that suggests you are doing something wrong and you need to revisit Groundhog Basic and consider upgrading to Groundhog Chronic (page 174).

Infectious disease can progress to serious illness, so always be mindful of the following nasties:

Table 18.2: Serious infections to be aware of

Symptom	Possible diagnosis	What to do
Severe headache which is worse with movement Often there is reflex muscle spasm which causes stiff neck Photophobia (can't bear light) Rash that does not blanch with pressure High fever and prostration Patient not 'with it' Child may be very irritable or restless	Meningitis or encephalitis Thankfully this is rare. During my 20 years of NHS general practice I diagnosed and admitted one case. I jabbed her with penicillin at home immediately and she did well. I would have an even lower threshold for diagnosing this in any person with a pre-existing brain problem, such as cerebral palsy or epilepsy	Urgent medical attention is needed. Penicillin may be lifesaving so if you have got any antibiotic in the house just take it! Get to hospital PDQ. **Note:** PDQ stands for 'Pretty Damn Quick'. This term was first used in *The Mighty Dollar*, a play by Benjamin E Woolf, and first performed in 1875 at New York's Park Theatre. The play's money-grabbing character, Judge Bardwell Stote, often used abbreviations like TTT – a 'tip-top time' – and GIC – 'goose is cooked'.
Stridor (noise from the upper airways on breathing in and out) and difficulty breathing	Epiglottitis – again, thankfully, this is rare and I have never seen a case	This is potentially fatal and needs urgent hospital treatment. Do not even try to look in the mouth to diagnose this because that can trigger airway obstruction.
Barking cough which sounds like a seal. Once heard, never forgotten!	Croup – which sounds much worse than it is. I have suffered croup. One good barking cough usually achieved a day off school	Many cases resolve once dairy products are cut out. Also worked for me. Dammit
Wheeze and shortness of breath 'Peak flow' drops below 50% of your personal best	Chest infections can flare asthma	Use the blue inhaler pretty much *ad lib* Take oral steroids and possibly antibiotics Get medical help
Patient obviously unwell with no local symptom or signs	Septicaemia (blood poisoning)	Get medical help

In addition, always look for progression of symptoms. If this occurs, as shown in Table 18.3, carry on with all above and add in what is recommended in the right-hand column. Remember, it is an arms race – you fight by throwing in additional troops, not replacing them.

Table 18.3: Action to take if symptoms develop further

If early symptoms progress to:	Consider possibility of:	...and treat with All THE ABOVE PLUS: (Note: Adult doses are given here so reduce proportionately for children (by weight))
Mucus from the nose becomes thick and green or brown Headache which is worse lying down	Acute sinusitis	I would prescribe doxycycline 100 mg twice daily for three days, then once daily until you can breathe normally through your nose Note that in children under the age of 8 doxycycline may stain their developing teeth so use cephalexin instead
Productive chesty cough with thick green or brown mucus	Acute bronchitis	Cephalexin 500 mg three times daily for at least a week or until two days after the symptoms have settled (those with poor immunity may need two weeks' worth)
Ear pain or deafness Irritable child	Ear infection	Cephalexin as above. Remember that many upper respiratory tract infections (URTIs) and catarrhal conditions are driven by allergies to **dairy** and **yeast**
Vomiting, diarrhoea, colicky tummy pain (i.e. it comes and goes), loss of appetite, feeling ghastly	Gastroenteritis	Do not suppress the symptoms as they are Nature's way of expelling microbes Do not feed the microbes: fast for at least 24 hours, possibly longer Keep hydrated: add ½ teaspoon (2.5 grams) of Sunshine salt (see page 238) to one litre of water and drink *ad lib*. If you cannot hydrate because of vomiting, then you will need an intravenous drip in hospital.
Back pain, pain on peeing, increased frequency of peeing, urgency	Urinary tract infection: Dip sticks to diagnose this are very helpful (page 220)	D-mannose (see page 218 – take 3 x 500 mg capsules one to three times daily) often works well. It prevents *E coli* from sticking to the lining of the urinary tract so that it is easily flushed out Potassium citrate (see page 219 for types and doses) reduces the symptoms If the symptoms do not improve within 36 hours I would prescribe an antibiotic, such as trimethoprim 200 mg twice daily, and continue for two days after the symptoms have settled

A very sore throat with swollen lymph nodes in the neck…	Tonsillitis	Gargle every hour with Lugol's iodine 12%, 4 drops in a small glass of water Penicillin 500 mg four times daily and continue for two days after the symptoms have settled Recurrent tonsillitis is typical of dairy allergy
…or, especially in a young person, consider	HHV4 (glandular fever) – always have a low threshold for suspecting this or HHV5 (cytomegalovirus) or HHV6 (roseola rash)	Gargle every hour with Lugol's iodine 12%, 4 drops in a small glass of water If the tonsillitis does not settle then get blood tests for HHV4, HHV5 and HHV6 I now know that these are such nasty, vicious viruses which so often trigger post-viral chronic fatigue syndrome that I would treat with valaciclovir 1 gram taken four times daily for at least a month, or until a good recovery Chinese skullcap is particularly good at killing herpes, but you need enough of it – at least 10 grams daily
Blistering lesions	Cold sores (HHV1) Genital herpes (HHV2) Chicken pox, shingles (HHV3)	Iodine ointment sufficient to stain yellow Topical antivirals are also helpful, such as aciclovir cream used *ad lib* Lysine 1 gram (1000 mg) taken three times daily is of proven benefit in preventing and treating HHVs A systemic antiviral, such as valaciclovir
Rashes which fade on contact – press a glass against the skin to see; essentially, these are 'allergy' reactions to virus	German measles Measles Scarlet fever Slapped cheek *Erythema multiforme* (allergy to *Herpes simplex*)	Rashes may look awful but are rarely serious; the basic package of treatment allows rapid recovery Iodine eye drops, such as povidone iodine 5%, are excellent for the conjunctivitis of measles
Rashes which do not fade on contact	These are due to bleeding under the skin and herald serious disease	Get professional help PDQ

If early symptoms progress to:	Consider possibility of:	...and treat with All THE ABOVE PLUS: (Note: Adult doses are given here so reduce proportionately for children (by weight))
Dental infections	Dental abscess or gingivitis: treat aggressively or you risk losing teeth	This is a powerful imperative to do a PK diet. Once you are PK-adapted, dental infections become a thing of the past (see Chapter 24, page 114) Co-amoxiclav 500/125 g three times daily and continue for two days after the symptoms have settled If no better in two days, add in metronidazole 400 mg three times daily and continue for two days after symptoms have settled Chew the capsules in the mouth to really hit the microbes – yes, this tastes awful!
Swollen cheeks with a hamster-like appearance	Mumps	Use iodine ointment *ad lib* over the swollen salivary glands to stain the skin yellow Generally there is little problem in girls or pre-pubertal boys Post-pubertal boys can get a nasty orchitis [inflamed testes]: this is a good reason not to have mumps vaccination which may simply postpone the age at which men get infected

Some health purists may criticise my use of antibiotics, but being old and experienced I have seen people either get nasty complications or die because antibiotics were withheld inappropriately. One death occurred locally when the GP diagnosed over the phone and did not prescribe antibiotics because his stoical patient 'just had 'flu'. My view is that with evolutionarily correct diets and lifestyles in place we are greatly protected against the potential malign effects of antibiotics. I would not like to practise medicine without ready access to such – they are the Exocet missiles of our modern armamentarium. However, the need for them should prompt one to re-examine the Groundhog interventions and whether they are being followed adequately.

Chronic or recurrent ENT infections

These ear, nose and throat infections include otitis media (inflammation of the middle ear), sinusitis, tonsillitis, laryngitis, croup and chest infections. Very often these are associated with allergy to dairy products. A tendency to such runs strongly in families – I do not think I have ever seen a dairy allergic who did not also have a first-degree relative similarly afflicted. Dairy products seem to encourage mucus and catarrh, which narrow airways and result in mouth breathing or noisy breathing. When infection gets a grip, we have all the inflammation symptoms of more mucus (blockage and deafness), sneezing, chesty cough, wheezing, pain, fever and general misery.

Antibiotics may be necessary to get rid of an established infection, but that must not be seen as the end of the story. Failure to apply at least Groundhog Basic (page 98) means that infection will return. Indeed, it is more likely to do so because infection results in inflammation with tissue damage and scarring. Scar tissue, being poorly perfused with blood, supplies microbes with a comfortable home in which to live – the body has unwittingly produced 'biofilm' (see page 231), a protective shield, for them.

The need for antibiotics, antifungals or antiviral drugs is symptomatic of Groundhog Basic not being done or Groundhog Acute (page 110) not being done soon enough or with sufficiently high or sufficiently regular doses of vitamin C and iodine. If these interventions are ineffective, then that points to immune suppression by some other pathology. If that is the case, investigate, possibly for chronic infection (see Chapters 27 and 28).

Table 18.4: Action to take for chronic or recurrent ENT infections

Diagnosis	Adult dose (halve the dose for a child)	Notes
Whatever the diagnosis, carry on with Groundhog Acute. You may need tens or hundreds of grams of vitamin C to achieve bowel tolerance	For acute one-off infection the duration of treatment can be for 48 hours after the symptoms have cleared	For chronic infection, the duration of treatment after symptoms have cleared should be much longer – certainly weeks (e.g. bronchiectasis), months for some (e.g. osteomyelitis, Epstein Barr ME), possibly years for others (e.g. TB, hepatitis C, HIV)
Otitis media	Cephalexin 500 mg three times daily	
Tonsillitis	Penicillin V 500 mg four times daily Gargle with Lugol's iodine 12% – 4 drops in a small glass of water *ad lib*. This is so effective because iodine is volatile and contact-kills viruses	Be aware that glandular fever may present with tonsillitis. The Epstein Barr virus (EBV) is very good at switching on allergy and so antibiotics should be avoided or a nasty drug reaction may ensue. Indeed, some doctors used to use this to diagnose EBV because amoxicillin almost invariably produces a nasty rash
Glandular fever	EBV is a particularly nasty virus and associated with so many other nasty conditions that I would now prescribe valaciclovir 1 gram taken four times daily to reduce the severity and duration of the illness Gargle with 5 drops Lugol's iodine 12% in a small glass of water *or* chew iodoral 12.5 mg tablets Smother swollen glands with iodine ointment	This often presents with tonsillitis Even if you do not know the cause of the tonsillitis, use iodine gargles Chinese skullcap 10 grams daily
Sinusitis	Doxycycline 100 mg twice daily Steam inhalation with a salt pipe of Lugol's iodine 12% (see above)	Acute and chronic sinusitis may also present with foul-smelling breath

Laryngitis	This is nearly always viral Vitamin C to bowel tolerance is very effective Steam inhalation with a salt pipe of Lugol's iodine 12% (see above)	
Croup	This is nearly always viral Steam inhalation with a salt pipe of Lugol's iodine 12% (see above) There seems to be a large element of viral allergy here and often a short course of steroids (e.g. prednisolone 5 mg x 4 tablets for two days) is very helpful	Cutting out the dairy products avoids recurrence
Conjunctivitis, iritis, indeed any eye infection	Iodine eye drops applied *ad lib* kill all eye infections – bacterial, viral and fungal	Conjunctivitis is a feature of measles – indeed, the virus accesses the human body through the eyes
Chest infections (bronchitis, pneumonias)	Cephalexin 500 mg three times daily (half this dose for a child) *or* Ciprofloxacin 500 mg twice daily Steam inhalation with a salt pipe of Lugol's iodine 12% (see above)	Often there is a large element of allergy, especially to dairy products and/or microbes
	When accompanied by respiratory distress, steroids may be essential – e.g. prednisolone 30 mg for three days, reducing the dose until the symptoms have settled	If you should ever need steroids, this is the most powerful imperative to do Groundhog in all its forms
Bronchiectasis	As above But many cases have an element of fungal infection – consider aspergillosis as a factor, in which case antifungals may be very helpful	Expert medical advice is needed but Groundhog Acute plus six weeks of itraconazole 100 mg daily, and possibly antibiotics, has the potential to cure bronchiectasis A salt pipe with Lugol's iodine 12% is a great weapon for all chronic respiratory conditions (see Chapter 10)
Sarcoidosis	This is an odd condition that has all the hall marks of chronic infection, but no clear causative microbe has been identified. *Propionibacterium acnes*, the acne bacterium, and mycobacteria (like the organism that causes TB) are contenders	Treat with Groundhog Chronic Steam inhalation with a salt pipe using Lugol's iodine 12% (see Chapter 10) Expert medical advice is needed

By putting in place these interventions we shall have become more cunning than the 'Professor' viruses of Chapter 4 fame (see page 22).

Blackadder: Baldrick, I have a very, very, very cunning plan.

Baldrick: Is it as cunning as a fox what used to be Professor of Cunning at Oxford University but has moved on and is now working for the UN at the High Commission of International Cunning Planning?

Blackadder: Yes it is.

Baldrick: Hmm... that's cunning.

From *Blackadder Back & Forth*

Finally, remember that many disease processes present with symptoms of inflammation. If symptoms grumble on, then there may well be a non-infectious cause (see our book *Sustainable Medicine – whistle blowing on 21st medical practice* for a starting point to treating chronic conditions).

Chapter 19

Measles, mumps, rubella, chicken pox and other such friendly immune programmers

Amicus protectio fortis – *strong protection by friends*

School Motto, Cedros School, Mexico City

We have evolved over millions of years with various infections. They are meant to be acquired in childhood and thereby render that child immune to that virus for the rest of its life. A major problem with mumps vaccination is that it does not confer lifelong immunity; the effect is to postpone the age at which the disease appears. I have seen several cases of mumps in adult men – they waddle into the surgery with tender testicles the size of a grapefruit. They can be ill for weeks and, indeed, risk sterility.

Story from Dr Myhill's surgery: Craig was attending a consultation for various matters, including having a lump on his left testicle checked out. It turned out to be a benign cyst. Anyway, picture the scene: Craig standing with his trousers and pants round his ankles and Sarah squatting in front of him. Without warning or even a knock on the door, a female secretary entered the consultation room and observed the scene before her. Quick as a flash Craig said, 'I have a sore throat and Sarah has told me that this is how doctors always examine sore throats, apparently.' Exit secretary! Sarah: Now you know he is a gentleman!

There is a general assumption that these viral infections are bad for us, but it is likely that they also do good. The immune system has to be exercised and programmed to work well. It is vital for it to learn to differentiate between self and non-self. We know a normal gut microbiome is essential to achieve this. Many childhood viruses are associated with cancers, neurological disease, autoimmunity and the like (see Chapter 2). How and when we acquire infection is critical to our immune response to such. We are ignorant of the fine checks and balances that have evolved to ensure survival and it seems to me to be nuts to interfere with these.

My personal view is that the training of our children's immune systems must mimic Nature. It is best to acquire these viral infections in childhood through natural exposures. This may well afford resistance to virally driven tumours. It may be no coincidence that the incidence of childhood leukaemia is rising.[63]

Groundhog Acute interventions prevent serious illness or complications from the childhood infections. Most importantly, Groundhog Acute is harmless. By contrast, vaccinations are potentially dangerous.

Table 19.1: Treatment of childhood viruses

Treatment of	With	And...
Measles	Groundhog Acute (see Chapter 17, page 110, and also Chapters 14 (page 84) and 18 (page 113)	Iodine eye drops for the inevitable conjunctivitis (see Chapter 10, page 64, for details) Iodine inhalations for the inevitable cough (see Chapter 10, page 64, for salt pipe method)
Mumps	Ditto. I have seen mumps pass in 24 hours with bowel-tolerance doses of vitamin C and topical iodine	Smother the swollen salivary glands with iodine ointment – enough to keep them yellow. Iodine is volatile so will penetrate the gland and contact-kill the virus
Rubella	Ditto	The sufferer must be kept socially isolated to avoid all women of child-bearing age. Rubella acquired during the first 12 weeks of pregnancy is teratogenic (causes fetal abnormalities). It is such a joke that women are not tested for rubella immunity until 12 weeks of pregnancy. This is far too late. Girls should be screened for rubella immunity at child-bearing age and vaccination considered at that point

Chicken pox (HHV3)	Ditto	Iodine ointment smothered on every spot. Keep them all yellow. This kills the virus directly and prevents secondary infection with other microbes
Shingles (HHV3)	Ditto Nasty – must treat aggressively	Topical iodine *ad lib* as above Antiviral drugs (see Chapter 22, page 211)
Scarlatina (allergic rash to *Streptococcus*)	Ditto	Penicillin may be necessary.
Molluscum contagiosum (sounds like a Harry Potter spell!) virus	Ditto	Not serious but looks bad Do not pick the lesions or you will end up with a scar; unpicked they heal without scarring Topical iodine ointment contact-kills the virus
Hand, foot and mouth (Coxsackie virus)	Ditto	Not serious but looks bad Topical iodine ointment.
Slapped cheek (Parvo virus)	Ditto	Not serious but looks bad
Pityriasis rosea (probably viral)	Ditto	Ditto

> You may notice the repetition of 'ditto' above? Ditto derives from a Tuscan dialect variant of the Italian *'detto'*, 'said', from the Latin *'dictus'*, 'said'.

The fact that I am repeating 'ditto' indicates that doing the basic things well is a good defence, and attack, against a wide variety of possible enemies. We have Groundhog Basic (Chapter 15), and then extra vitamin C (Chapter 9) and iodine (Chapter 10) plus the immune-supporting herbals (Chapter 13) and then for specific infections we add in specific attackers.

Chapter 20

Acute gut infections:
diarrhoea and vomiting

I have tried to lift France out of the mud. But she will return to her errors and vomitings. I cannot prevent the French from being French.
Charles de Gaulle (22 November 1890 – 9 November 1970)

Charles de Gaulle was perhaps wrong in wanting to stop the French from returning to her vomitings… certainly, in the case of disease, it is undesirable to suppress the symptoms of diarrhoea and vomiting. These symptoms are signs that the body is fighting an infection and it should be left to do so. But there are things that we can and should do to help.

Acute gastroenteritis is an important defence mechanism against pathogens and poisons. The main symptoms of vomiting and/or diarrhoea should not be inhibited by medications for obvious reasons. Do not be tempted to dive in with symptom-suppressing drugs; this may result in short-term gain but risks long-term pain.

Groundhog Acute (page 110) should be applied. Importantly, no food at all should be given until the symptoms have settled – this takes at least 24 hours (and it takes three days for the gut to heal fully). Any food simply feeds microbes. Of course, fluids are essential. These must be given in balance with essential salts. This is where Sunshine salt (page 238) is so helpful – it is a near physiological balance of all essential trace minerals. It is far superior to any other rehydrating fluid currently available. Make up a solution of 5 grams of Sunshine salt (a teaspoonful) in one litre of water, so providing a 0.5% solution. Drink this *ad lib*. The main problem arises if vomiting is prolonged and oral rehydration not possible. In this event, hospital admission for intravenous fluids is essential and may be life-saving.

Indeed, acute dehydration is the mechanism of death in cholera, which is one of the greatest killers of humans throughout history. Interestingly, cholera explains why the cystic fibrosis gene, present in one in 16 of the population, has survived. Heterozygotes (carriers of just one CF gene) have impaired chloride transport, so they do not dehydrate so quickly when they get cholera and so survive.

It may be impossible in acute gastroenteritis to ascertain bowel tolerance for vitamin C because one has diarrhoea already, but this is no reason not to use it. I would suggest 10 grams of vitamin C every hour for at least four cycles. This will contact-kill and detoxify the majority of gut pathogens and poisons. Then continue with rehydrating fluids only until the symptoms abate. If you are keto-adapted (see page 234), you should feel much better very quickly. It is the people who run on carbs who feel hypoglycaemic and are tempted to snack or drink fruit juice. Such temptation must be resisted as any sugar simply feeds the pathogens and risks chronic disease.

After a dose of gastroenteritis, the levels of friendly microbes in the gut will be low. This is when you need to feed them with a PK diet (page 234). Discourage the unfriendlies with fermented foods. Back to Groundhog Basic (or, as in my case, because I am old, Groundhog Chronic (page 174).) (*And* in my case also – Craig.)

A final note is never to underestimate acute gut infections. In the West we have become blasé about these, as we have about many infections, because of the false promise of antibiotics. As mentioned previously, antibiotics are a very useful line of attack and I would not want to practise medicine without them, but they are far from giving us all our answers. We must box clever and use all the other weapons at our disposal, as described in this book, if we are to stay ahead of the game in this arms race.

Remember that across the world, diarrhoeal disease is the second leading cause of death in children under five years old. It was a possible cause of death of Alaric, the Visigoth Chieftain who sacked Rome in AD 410, and who had previously survived several brutal wounds during many vicious battles. Malaria is another possible cause of death of Alaric, touted by many, but whatever the truth of the matter, he was floored by a microbe, invisible to the human eye, having fought and beaten the might of the Roman Army and its thousands of legionaries. A lesson to us all!

Chapter 21

Urinary tract infections (UTIs)

My love for you burns deeper than my urinary tract infection…

Internet meme

However, UTIs are no joke. They must always be taken seriously, monitored and, if sufficient defences, such as Groundhog Acute are not properly in place, then they must be treated promptly, otherwise one risks a kidney infection. The key is to have Groundhog Basic, and possibly Groundhog Chronic, in place effectively for long enough and then UTIs will become a thing of the past.

We are seeing epidemics of cystitis and urethritis. Often a microbe cannot be identified on swabs or urine samples, but antibiotics are prescribed. This may be effective clinically in the short term, but so often I see progression to recurrent and then persistent symptoms of perineal pain and inflammation, with disturbances of micturition (urination). Interstitial cystitis, or in men, prostatitis or epididymitis, may be diagnosed. What is going on?

My working hypothesis, which has served well over the past 35 years, has three strands.

1. **Sensitisation**: First, infection with a microbe results in subsequent sensitisation to such. Diagnosis of a UTI is made when a urine sample contains at least 10,000 microbes per millilitre (ml) of urine. Some months later, identical symptoms may arise when an MSU (mid-stream specimen of urine test) is 'negative' – that is, there are fewer than 10,000 microbes per ml. In this event, the patient has become 'allergic' to that microbe, with inflammation (and therefore symptoms) being

switched on with perhaps just 500 microbes per ml. Every time there is infection and inflammation, there is tissue damage with the formation of scar tissue. This scar tissue is never as well perfused with blood as normal tissue and so forms a comfortable environment in which terrorist microbes can make themselves at home. We are starting to lose the arms race.

2. **Antibiotic resistance and proliferation:** Secondly, once one microbe makes itself at home in scar tissue, others will follow. Either the existing microbe or the new kid on the block can cause infection, and each has different antibiotic sensitivities, so successive rounds of antibiotic treatment of symptom flares become less and less effective.

3. **Bacterial translocation**: We have to ask, from where do the infective microbes come? In women, with their short urethras, some come from below upwards – sex and baths. Studies[64] suggest that bath water does get into the female bladder an extraordinary 30% of the time! However, my view is that the majority of microbes come from the fermenting gut. The idea here is that a high-carb diet allows microbes to ferment in the upper gut (stomach and small intestine) which should be pretty much sterile. These microbes, being miniscule, easily get from the gut into the bloodstream. This is called 'bacterial translocation' (see below), but of course yeasts and other microbes translocate too. They are excreted through the kidneys. Humans have been doing this for millions of years. However, each fermenting microbe has its own preferred food; we have learned to deal with those which ferment fibres, but not those which feed off sugars and starches – now in abundance in modern Western diets, whereas previously these would have been scarce sources of food. Therefore, because of our modern Western diets, we have more microbial translocation than ever before, and this is switching on the immune system and driving many pathologies.

Treatment of all the above

For an acute infection, apply Groundhog Acute (page 110). That may be all that is required. For chronic symptoms apply Groundhog Chronic (page 174).

Consider using antimicrobials such as:

- **D mannose:** This is the best natural antibiotic for UTIs. To infect, microbes first have to stick to the lining of the urinary tract (otherwise they are easily washed out by urine). D mannose coats the sticky paws of the microbes, meaning that the microbe cannot stick to the urinary tract lining, and so they are easily flushed away. This only works for the *E coli* microbe, but this is a common cause of UTIs. The dose is 500 mg every two to three hours, continued for at least three days after symptoms have settled.
- **Berberine** works in a similar way to D mannose. It is the active ingredient in goldenseal and a reasonable dose would be 1 gram taken three times daily.
- **Potassium/magnesium citrate** often relieves symptoms. Interestingly this is also a great treatment for preventing calcium oxalate renal stones.[65]

All these three can be taken at the same time. Indeed, the more ways one can hit infection the better.

If you are still struggling, then antibiotics may become necessary, such as trimethoprim 200 mg twice daily to be continued for three days after symptoms have settled. But remember, the need for antibiotics is a symptom of not applying Groundhog sufficiently well. Again, the principles are:

- starve the little wretches out with a PK diet;
- kill 'em with vitamin C.

Should you need any extra incentive to do this, remember many tumours are driven by chronic infection. Prostate cancer candidates include xenotrophic murine retrovirus (XMRV – also implicated in CFS/ME), trichomonas (an STD), herpes viruses, *Propionibacterium acnes* (the microbe that causes acne) and probably others. Bladder cancer is more likely in people with in-dwelling catheters, which are invariably infected.

By winning battles now (against chronic infections), you will avoid the need to fight bigger battles later (against cancers). Don't appease, and don't feed the fermenting gut. As Churchill said, of different battles and different appeasements:

An appeaser is one who feeds a crocodile, hoping it will eat him last.

Sir Winston Leonard Spencer-Churchill, KG OM CH TD PCC DL FRS RA

(30 November 1874 – 24 January 1965)

Chapter 22

Skin infections

Your birthday suit accounts for about 15% of your total body weight and is replaced every month. Some sources estimate that dead skin comprises about a billion tons of dust in the Earth's atmosphere.[66] In literature, we have phrases such as 'goosebumps' (indicating excitement or fear; in the US – 'gooseflesh') and 'skin crawl' (indicating disgust) whereby emotional states are conveyed via the 'feel' of our skin. Helen of Troy's face was famously 'fair of skin' and it was her face that 'launched a thousand ships':

Was this the face that launch'd a thousand ships

And burnt the topless towers of Ilium?

Sweet Helen, make me immortal with a kiss.
> Christopher Marlowe (6 February 1564 – 30 May 1593)
> *The Tragical History of Doctor Faustus* referring to 'Helen of Greece'

Skin then is important not just as a barrier against a hostile world. Helen's fair skin started a ten-year war, but here we shall concentrate on the importance of skin in our own personal war – the arms race going on inside our bodies.

The skin is a vital, natural barrier against infection which, if breached, allows microbes in that may infect. This is where good hygiene and dressings are essential. In short, our skin is a wall in the arms race.

Cuts, grazes, wounds, burns, spots, active eczema and other skin breaches

If suffering from any of these:
- Clean as best you can, ideally with copious amounts of Lugol's iodine 12% (approximately 10 ml in 500 ml of water), salty water (1 teaspoon of salt in 500 ml of water) or vitamin C (1 teaspoon in 500 ml of water) to physically wash out any dirt or other such contaminants. If you are caught out in the wild, then peeing over and scrubbing the wound works well too – urine is near sterile. If there is any hint of foreign bodies, such as splinters, gravel or ingrained dirt, then surgical treatment may be necessary as wounds never heal if foreign bodies remain present.
- Allow the wound to dry.
- Once dry, smother it with iodine 10% ointment. You can see the yellow stain of iodine – keep it yellow! (Iodine is particularly suited to skin problems because, being volatile, it penetrates skin and flesh extremely well. Furthermore, by contrast with many other disinfectants, iodine is not toxic to human cells, so healing and repair progress unabated.) Then keep the wound dressed until the skin heals over to prevent further contamination.

Boils and abscesses

Now we must turn our attention to boils and abscesses, including styes (eyelash infection), paronychia (nail-bed infection), impetigo, erysipelas, folliculitis (hair follicle infection), pilonidal sinus, ischiorectal (bum) abscess and other nasty inflamed lumps.

Thou art a boil, a plague sore, an embossed carbuncle in my corrupted blood.
King Lear by William Shakespeare (1564 – 23 April 1616)
(Lear says this of the eldest of his three daughters, Goneril, in Act 2 Scene 4)

We now know that Lear was wrong – boils and the like are not caused by daughters, however evil they may be, but rather they are largely caused by *Staphylococcus aureus*. Many of us have staph on our skin and up our noses – this microbe is impossible to avoid. The key to prevention is to improve the defences; it is back to Groundhog Basic. Sugar is clearly an important player here – diabetes, for example, often presents with recurrent skin infections. Avoid sugar!

- At the first sign of any abscess or boil, apply Groundhog Acute together with topical iodine ointment 10% *ad lib*. This alone may get rid of the problem.
- If the infection is around your eyes or nose, then take this very seriously; there is potential for the infection to spread back into the brain and cause a cavernous sinus thrombosis. Antibiotics are essential protection against this nasty possibility.
- However, once a boil is maturing, avoid antibiotics. If they are effective, the boil will stop growing and you will be left with a permanent lump, an 'antibiotic-oma', which may cause problems in the future. Instead, poultice or hot bathe the boil to draw it to a head and then discharge itself. There is nothing more satisfying than to see the gungy contents expelled, with instant relief.

Horses are occasionally afflicted by pus in the foot, known as 'gravel'. The pressure of the boil within the hard hoof chamber renders them acutely lame. As the farrier finds the source, he is hit in the eye by a stream of pressurised pus. This is accompanied by a sigh of relief from the horse and the smiles of any on-lookers – a real champagne moment! James Herriot would follow this up by packing the cavity with iodine crystals, then adding turpentine; the explosion that followed drove the iodine deep into the infected cavity but as importantly produced an impressive purple cloud and an equally impressive reaction even in the most dour of Yorkshire farmers!

Cellulitis

This is a potentially lethal extension of the infections above. If a local infection has not been adequately dealt with, then a red line will be seen streaking up to the local lymph node, which will swell to a painful hot lump as it fights infection. This is a prelude to septicaemia and must always be taken seriously. In addition to applying all the above and Groundhog Acute, systemic antibiotics are essential, possibly even given intravenously. Urgent, professional attention is necessary.

Acne

Acne is a miserable affliction that scars the life of sufferers when they are at their most vulnerable. It afflicts up to 95% of adolescents in Western societies. By contrast in a

study of 1200 Kitavan subjects examined, including 300 aged 15-25 years, no case
of acne (grade 1 with multiple comedones or grades 2-4) was observed. Of 115 Aché
subjects examined (including 15 aged 15-25 years) over 843 days, no case of active acne
(grades 1-4) was observed.[67] (Kitava is one of the four major islands in the Trobriand
Islands archipelago group of the Solomon Sea, located in Milne Bay Province of south
eastern Papua New Guinea. The Kitavan diet is uninfluenced by the modern Western
diet and comprises an abundance of foods that have a low glycaemic index rating. There
is also practically no diabetes, cardiovascular disease leading to stroke or congestive
heart failure, dementia or high blood pressure among native Kitavans. The Aché are an
indigenous people of Paraguay; they are hunter-gatherers.) This tells us that Western
diets and lifestyles are to blame and explains why the PK (paleo-ketogenic) diet is
highly effective. From my experience I know there are at least two causes of acne –
carbohydrates (probably mediated by the fermenting gut), and allergy to dairy products.
Groundhog Basic is highly effective at curing acne. Of course, I am applying this to that
age of patient least willing to take advice from an old crone like me. I have a rule of
thumb that I can do very little to help those between the ages of 14 and 24 because they
already know all there is to know about Life. However, vanity is a powerful motivating
influence and I have a few notable successes in persuasion.

I am not young enough to know everything.
The Admirable Crichton by JM Barrie (9 May 1860 – 19 June 1937),
and Oscar Wilde (16 October 1854 – 30 November 1900) – attribution uncertain.

A few find their acne worsened by this regime. I suspect this is a detox effect. The clue
can be found in the skin reaction to organochlorine poisoning – so-called chloracne. This
produces similar lesions by an unknown mechanism. I have had several patients who
have been chemically poisoned, developed acne whilst detoxing with heat treatments
(such as sauna-ing), have persisted with treatment regardless and eventually found the
acne reaction resolved. I can only explain this by a reaction to toxins being excreted
through the skin.

Some people being treated with vitamin B12 by injection, and indeed iodine, also
get an acne reaction. Both B12 and iodine are good at mobilising toxins from the body.
Again, this resolves with time if the sufferer is prepared to put up with the acne for a few
weeks.

The key point to remember is that conventional, doctor-driven treatments of acne are potentially dangerous:

1. Long-term antibiotics: In those eating Western, carbohydrate-based diets, these have massive potential to disrupt the gut microbiome.
2. The Pill: This is one of my most hated medications. The Pill is immunosuppressive, induces metabolic syndrome with all its complications, may lead to promiscuity with all its complications (see Chapter 23) and is growth promoting, so carcinogenic. The Pill often causes depression and I suspect is a major risk factor for suicide.
3. Ro-accutane: This is a toxic drug closely allied to those used in cancer chemotherapy. I have seen three suicides in teenagers who have used this drug. I think it also a major risk factor for chronic fatigue syndrome.

The infecting organism of acne is *Propionibacterium acnes*. This same microbe is also implicated in some cases of post-operative infection, prosthesis failure, arthritis, prostate cancer and sarcoidosis. Treatment of course is Groundhog Basic. That should be all that is necessary. The young sufferer may moan and groan at me, but as my patients so often hear me say: 'My job is to get you better, not to entertain you.'

> In his *Satires*, Juvenal (1st century AD – 2nd century AD) wrote of *'Panem et circenses'*, meaning 'bread and circuses', referring to the basic needs and desires of the 'plebs' — food and entertainment. He was wrong about the bread, unless he was referring to PK bread (see our book *The PK Cookbook*.) He was right about the entertainment, but that is not my job!

Body odour (BO)

Sweat has almost no smell. It is simply blood but without the large bits like cells and proteins. It does contain sugar, and the higher the blood sugar, the more sugar there is in sweat. This provides a free lunch for microbes on the skin. They love moist conditions and so thrive in armpits, tits and other naughty bits.

Sarah is a poet and I didn't know it! She speaks in rhyme all of the time – Craig

If your microbes ferment this sugar to something that smells nasty, then you too will smell nasty. BO is part of the metabolic syndrome of Westerners eating carbohydrate-based diets. Treatment of course is Groundhog Basic, perhaps combined with topical iodine.

To illustrate the above point, there have been interesting experiments done to change the offending microbes. The sufferer has plastered his smelly areas with antiseptics to kill the indigenous flora. He has then received a sweaty donation, ideally from a non-stinking family member, and thereby recolonised offending departments. The problem has been greatly relieved. The prospect of this procedure has provided useful clinical leverage for those reluctant to embrace Groundhog.

If you need to be further persuaded, consider this. The conventional treatment is to use deodorant. This works because it contains aluminium which kills all microbes. Unfortunately, it also kills humans – aluminium is well absorbed through the skin and causes Alzheimer's disease. It may contribute to the development of breast cancer and may explain why cancers are more common in the upper outer quadrant of the breast.[68]

Tinea, ringworm, athlete's foot, jock itch

The causes of these common fungal problems are the same as for BO – a high-carb diet feeding microbes. So is the treatment (see above and also Chapter 26, Fungi and yeasts).

Shingles (*Varicella zoster* virus, human herpes virus 3 (HHV3))

Shingles is not really a skin infection but an infection of the nerves which manifest with a nasty rash. It is caused by the chicken pox virus. One has to have had prior infection with chicken pox. This explains why you can catch chicken pox from someone with shingles, but not the other way around. The virus then lives in the spinal cord and comes to life if the body's defences go down. Indeed, when I see shingles in any person I wonder why – is there an under-lying nasty, such as a tumour?

Not only is shingles very painful, but there is also a risk of developing a long-standing

post-herpetic neuralgia. (I think of this as viral allergy.) Post-herpetic neuralgia affects nerve fibres and skin, causing burning pain that lasts long after the rash and blisters of shingles have disappeared. Shingles must be treated aggressively. In order of priority:
- Groundhog Basic and Acute
- Smother the rash with iodine ointment *ad lib* so the area is constantly stained yellow
- Take antivirals, such as aciclovir 800 mg five times daily, until the rash has healed. This may mean a few weeks of treatment, but this is important in order to reduce the risk of post-herpetic neuralgia.

Cold Sores (human herpes virus 1 (HHV1))

HHV1 manifests with painful blisters on the lips. Again, treat and prevent this with Groundhog and topical iodine ointment *ad lib*.

Varicose (or venous) ulcers

Typically, varicose ulcers present in older people, initially with thin and discoloured skin, sometimes associated with varicose veins and thread veins, over the shin and ankle, which then breaks down and refuses to heal. I think there are at least three strands to the treatment of venous ulcers:

1. Pooling of blood in the legs. When the primitive ape stood up this made him a better hunter. He could run down his prey and have arms available to hurl stones and spears, but, after years of being vertical, it brought certain disadvantages – poor drainage of the sinus cavities, a tendency to groin hernias, a tendency to incontinence and a high-pressure system in the lower half of the body, with potential to cause piles and varicose veins. This high-pressure system is partly responsible for varicose ulcers. Venous blood pools and toxins are not cleared. The return of blood to the heart through the veins can be massively improved by graduated pressure tights; the idea here is that the compression must be greatest in the toe and foot and least at the top of the leg. With any exercise, the venous blood is massaged away and this prevents stagnation. The fit of the stocking must be perfect – obviously if it is tighter at the top than at the bottom the situation will be made worse. Get yourself a pair of tights from www.daylong.co.uk. If you are

sitting down, then your legs must be up (ideally at the level of your heart so the venous pressure in your legs is almost zero – a recliner chair is a great start). If you are not sitting down, then wear tights and move!

2. Allergy to microbes from the fermenting gut. Before the skin breaks down, the pre-ulcer skin will show all the hallmarks of inflammation.
3. Chronic infection. As soon as the skin is breached, the microbes move in and make themselves at home. They find a warm free lunch of sugar and moisture.

Once the mechanism of damage is clear, treatment follows logically. In order of priority:
- Groundhog Basic (for the fermenting gut)
- Graduated pressure stockings, recliner chair and exercise
- Treat open ulcers as above for all skin breaches, applying topical iodine for starters. Antibiotics may be needed to get ahead of the game
- Continue with Groundhog for life, otherwise the problem will simply recur for the same reasons that it arose in the first place.

Finally, be mindful that if the ulcer is not healing despite all the above, then it should be biopsied; sometimes there is malignant change.

Multiresistant *Staphylococcus aureus* (MRSA)

MRSA is a particular problem in hospitals where there are open wounds. Hospitals create a perfect storm where none of the Groundhog imperatives are in place and antibiotics are heavily used. This is an ideal habitat for growing antibiotic-resistant strains of microbe. Sick patients are fed junk food diets, high in sugar and refined carbohydrate. Vitamin supplements are often forbidden. Relatives are encouraged to bring in fruit, but fruit is a bag of sugar and feeds microbes. These disastrous conditions occur just when the need for a healthy diet and lifestyle is greatest. Hospitals are dangerous places to be.

In hospital, the emphasis needs to be on prevention. If you find yourself stuck in hospital, do not permit anyone to touch your wound without first seeing them either wash their hands or don surgical gloves. Do your best to apply Groundhog. After I broke my neck and was stuck in a neurosurgical unit, I was saved from starvation (the hospital 'food' was inedible) by my lovely daughter who appeared with good food, supplements and water.

No microbe, including MRSA, is resistant to iodine. Use iodine ointment *ad lib* as above. Remember the work of Dr Marik described in Chapter 9 (page 60). This consultant reduced mortality from septicaemia from 40% to 1% by adding intravenous vitamin C into his regimens. My guess that if all antibiotic prescriptions were combined with Groundhog, antibiotic resistance would become a thing of the past.

And now we move onto sex...

Chapter 23

Sexually transmitted diseases (STDs)

The body has excellent defences against inhaled and swallowed pathogens but very poor defences against STDs. The best defence is abstinence but if this were carried through, the species would rapidly go extinct. So, to ensure our survival, powerful reward systems have been factored in – we call these love, lust, passion and orgasm. Delightful as they are, these reward systems result in appalling risk-taking behaviour. This is driven by hormones that put us into a state of insanity where we do mad things. We all recognise this and, indeed, great works of Art result from such!

Rosalind in *As You Like It* states that:

Love is merely a madness and, I tell you, deserves as well a dark house and a whip as madmen do, and the reason why they are not so punished and cured is that the lunacy is so ordinary that the whippers are in love, too.

William Shakespeare (1564 – 23 April 1616)

There are countless other such examples of the insanity of lovers from antiquity to modern times. But, money talks – every year, Hollywood releases about 600 films and makes about $10 billion in profit whereas 13,000 porn films are released each year, netting close to $15 billion in profit.

We worsen these risks with the Pill, which may protect from pregnancy but increases the risk of STDs being acquired and getting established.

Thankfully, in the West, we have in place well-organised systems for diagnosing, contact-tracing and treating STDs. If you have put yourself at risk, then you must use a 'Special Clinic' to get diagnosed and effectively treated and then good contact-tracing must be done to identify others at risk. It is beyond the scope of this book to detail the conventional antibiotic treatment of STDs – just be sure you get professional help. However, all such treatments will be far more effective with Groundhog in place. You may be lucky and have a disease that can be eliminated with a course of antibiotics – such as syphilis, gonorrhoea, trichomonas or bacterial vaginosis. However, many STDs, such as *Chlamydia*, HIV, hepatitis, genital herpes, human papilloma virus, and syphilis, move into a chronic phase. This may start with a 'flu like illness and then microbes spread further to cause systemic inflammation, organic disease and perhaps organ failure.

You may well choose to continue Groundhog Chronic for life to protect yourself from the serious potential consequences of microbes driving pathology.

Genital herpes HHV2

This infection, once acquired, is for life, although repeat outbreaks are usually shorter and less severe than the first. Treat as:
- Groundhog Basic, possibly Groundhog Chronic
- Iodine ointment *ad lib* – to stain and keep stained yellow.

I make no apologies for sounding like a bore. Once again, my job is to get you better, not to entertain you! Actually, I am quite proud of myself in this chapter because I have managed to avoid using sexual innuendo, but it was difficult I tell you, very difficult!

Chapter 24

Dental infections and mouth ulcers

Get up from your chair, trot through to the bathroom and stand in front of a mirror with a bright light. Open your mouth. You can see with your own eyes if you are losing the arms race.

- Look at your teeth. Feel the surface with your tongue. They should be clean and smooth as glass. If you are not sure, use disclosing fluid which stains dental plaque purple. Dental plaque is biofilm – behind this lie colonies of bacteria eating into your teeth and infecting your gums. More teeth are lost to gum disease than any other mechanism. Once there, microbes spill over into the bloodstream and drive pathology, especially arterial disease.
- Look at your gums. Are they swollen or receded, indicating microbial damage?
- Look at your tongue. It should be pink and clean. Scrape your tongue with your teeth; there should be no crud – any such is made up of microbial colonies.
- Look inside your cheeks. Again, they should be pink and clean. White patches may represent yeast infection or pre-malignant change called 'leucoplakia'. Are there any ulcers or blisters?

Whilst looking, have you any dental amalgam? See Chapter 12 for the problems associated with this and the danger of dentists.

If any of the above problems are present, you will be at risk of infection – local to the mouth or distal (elsewhere in the body).

Dental decay, tooth abscesses, coated tongue and gum disease

These problems are universal in people eating Western diets. All these conditions can be abolished by eating the PK (paleo-ketogenic) diet. It is gum disease that results in all the miseries of rotten teeth, extractions and false teeth. Dentists have the power to do great good but also great harm. Dental amalgam fillings leak toxic metals, especially mercury, from the day they are put in. They cannot resist using fluoride, a highly toxic element which bioaccumulates in the body and does little to reduce tooth decay, but is neurotoxic, carcinogenic and damaging to the thyroid and bones.

The effect of fluoridation of water is even more stark than fluoride in toothpaste. In their medical paper, 'Water Fluoridation: A Critical Review of the Physiological Effects of Ingested Fluoride as a Public Health Intervention',[69] which reviewed all available research, Stephen Peckham and Niyi Awofeso concluded that:

- There was only 'modest' benefit to dental health.
- All but one study reviewed suggested that high fluoride content in water might negatively affect cognitive development.
- In a 2005 study, it was found that 47% of children living in a New Delhi neighbourhood with an average water fluoride level of 4.37 ppm have evidence of clinical hypothyroidism attributable to fluoride. They found borderline low FT3 levels among all children exposed to fluoridated water. 'FT3' is 'Free T3' and is the active thyroid hormone. Borderline low levels indicate that fluoridation of water has disrupted thyroid function.
- Dental fluorosis, also called mottling of tooth enamel, is a developmental disturbance of dental enamel caused by the consumption of excess fluoride during tooth development. About 41% of children in the United States, where water has been fluoridated at an average level of 1 ppm, have varying degrees of dental fluorosis, with levels of over 50% in some fluoridated areas.
- Population-based studies strongly suggest that chronic fluoride ingestion is a possible cause of uterine cancer and bladder cancer; there may also be a link with osteosarcoma.

Back to the microbes. The main offender is *Streptococcus mutans*. It is sensitive to neem, so neem toothpaste, sticks and mouthwash are all helpful, and neem avoids the need to put fluoride in your mouth.

Strep mutans is sensitive to amoxicillin and this is the first-line antibiotic for dental abscesses. Indeed, my view is that this antibiotic, in the form of co-amoxiclav 500/125 g three times daily, should be available over the counter so that people can self-treat at the first sign of dental pain and prevent progression to an abscess and possible tooth loss. If this does not do the trick, then metronidazole 400 mg three times daily sends the cavalry in. Do not rely on antibiotics in the long term – the infection will return for the very reasons you got it in the first place. The need for antibiotics is a wake-up call to at least do Groundhog Basic (page 98).

Finally, to illustrate the importance of eating the PK diet as an overarching protection against dental infections, consider the paper[70] which concludes that:

- 'Data from 34 early European skeletons indicate that the transition from hunter-gatherer to farming shifted the oral microbial community to a disease-associated configuration' – that is, eating a more carbohydrate-based diet encouraged the growth of bad bugs.
- '…hunter-gatherer groups displayed fewer caries- and periodontal disease-associated taxa' – that is, less tooth decay and disease was associated with a more 'PK-style' diet.
- 'Farming populations also displayed more periodontal disease-associated taxa, including *P. gingivalis*, *Tannerella* and *Treponema*, than hunter-gatherers' – that is again, eating a more carbohydrate-based diet encouraged the growth of bad bugs.

Fascinatingly, there has been recent research, reported in the *National Geographic*,[71] that teeth found in the 2000-year-old pre-Mesolithic cemetery at Al Khiday 2 (in modern-day Sudan) showed very little tooth decay, despite this being a farming society. One would have expected high levels of tooth decay due to the high-carbohydrate diet. Further investigation uncovered the answer to this apparent anomaly – this community of people also ate purple nutsedge, which has strong antimicrobial qualities. It is unsure how this habit of eating this noxious weed came about because it is foul-tasting (perhaps it was a chance happening and the general antimicrobial properties became apparent), but whatever, its presence in the diet of these ancient people most likely helped to lessen the amount of tooth decay.

Fortunately, we don't have to eat a noxious weed to avoid tooth decay; the recipes detailed in *The PK Cookbook* are delicious, and moreover, the PK diet prevents all types of dental infections, not just tooth decay. Yippee!

Treatment of any mouth infection

The mouth is at the interface of the inside and outside worlds and so ulcers have many possible causes, such as allergy to foods, nutritional deficiency, chronic infection or autoimmunity. If infected, Groundhog Basic (page 98) may do the trick, and topical iodine or vitamin C may be effective. I suggest chewing an iodoral tablet (more convenient than Lugol's 12%, 4 drops in water) or a *neutral form of vitamin C, 1 gram 30 minutes after food, and holding it in your mouth for as long as you can. It may take a few weeks to get rid of dental plaque with this regime.

Footnote: A form of vitamin C that is pH neutral (7) is important to avoid eroding dental enamel, which may occur if ascorbic acid is held in the mouth for long periods of time. So, for example, use magnesium ascorbate, which is non-acidic.

Chapter 25

Fermenting gut
You are on the slippery slope:
chronic disease is upon you

The upper gut (oesophagus, stomach and small intestine) should be nearly sterile for the digestion and absorption of fat, protein and micronutrients. It may contain a few grams of microbes. By contrast, the lower gut (large intestine) is a fermenting gut and holds kilograms of microbes to deal with fibre. Problems arise with high-carbohydrate diets; such diets overwhelm our ability to digest and absorb these carbohydrates quickly, so microbes move in to ferment this carbohydrate load. This results in an upper fermenting gut, which is highly abnormal (but unfortunately increasingly common), and many chronic systemic infections start with this process.

The upper fermenting gut

By 'the upper fermenting gut' I mean, microbes living in the lumen of the upper gut ferment foods where no such fermentation should take place. There is much more detail about this in our books *Sustainable Medicine – whistle blowing on 21st century medical practice* and *Diagnosis and Treatment of Chronic Fatigue Syndrome and Myalgic Encephalitis – it's mitochondria, not hypochondria*, but in a nutshell, these upper-gut fermenting microbes cause problems for several reasons. The clinical picture may be called 'irritable bowel syndrome', but remember, this is not a diagnosis, just a description!

Table 25.1: Symptoms of fermentation in the upper gut

Symptoms of upper fermenting gut	Mechanism – which applies to all microbial fermentation	Resulting in...
Burping and bloating	Results from the gas produced by fermentation of sugar (and digested sugar from carbs) by yeast. Burping is a cardinal symptom of upper fermenting gut.	Abdominal distension
Acid reflux	Results from the hypochlorhydria (reduced stomach acid) of the upper fermenting gut. Insufficient stomach acid means the stomach cannot empty because the plug hole of the stomach that separates it from the small intestine only opens up when a certain acidity has been achieved. Poor emptying plus low-grade inflammation results in reflux and oesophagitis.	Reflux damages the lining of the oesophagus so microbes can invade. This causes oesophagitis and possibly the narrowing of the oesophagus, and drives oesophageal cancer... and, I suspect, many other bowel tumours.
Foggy brain	Results from the toxins produced by fermentation. If there is fermentation in the upper gut due to yeast, almost invariably there is also fermentation due to bacteria. There may be a cocktail of products of this fermentation, such as ethyl alcohol, butyl alcohol and propyl alcohol. (These are initially metabolised in the liver to become toxic aldehydes.) Also, hydrogen sulphide, ammonia, nitric oxide, D lactate and more.	If the liver is overwhelmed by products of fermentation, then alcohol, D lactate and hydrogen sulphide spill over into the systemic bloodstream to cause the symptom of foggy brain, and probably foggy immune system also.
Carbohydrate cravings	Alcohol stimulates insulin release directly; this drops blood sugar levels, with an out-pouring of adrenalin and so-called 'hypoglycaemia' attacks.	Sufferers know that they can relieve their symptoms by eating carbs and so feed the very microbes that are causing the problem. It turns us into addicts! I see this as a clever evolutionary ploy by gut microbes to make their host eat the foods they wish to ferment.
Malabsorption	Microbes consume raw materials which are meant to feed you and me.	Lack of nutrition will result in immune suppression and fatigue.

Symptoms of upper fermenting gut	Mechanism – which applies to all microbial fermentation	Resulting in...
Fatigue	Microbes ferment to produce toxic substances, such as alcohol, D lactate and hydrogen sulphide, all of which have to be dealt with by the liver. This is greatly demanding of energy and raw materials. Indeed, the liver consumes more energy than the brain and heart combined.	This kicks a metabolic hole in the energy bucket to result in the symptom of fatigue and, again, immune suppression.
Allergy reactions in the gut, with pain and inflammation	The immune system is activated in the gut against yeast and/or bacteria...	...possibly leading to inflammatory bowel disease.
Allergy/ inflammation reactions at distal sites (elsewhere in the body)	The immune system is activated in the body against yeast and/or bacteria; this has the potential to switch on allergy, autoimmunity and chronic inflammation.	This can lead to interstitial cystitis, urticaria, asthma, migraine, arthritis, venous ulcers, psoriasis, eczema and many autoimmune diseases.

Treatment of the fermenting gut is with Groundhog Acute (page 110):
- starve the little wretches out with a PK diet and
- kill 'em with vitamin C.

Use this as a practice run for what you will need to do when you pick up an acute cold or 'flu. This combination is highly effective. Once you are ahead of the game you can return to Groundhog Basic (page 98).

Let us pay good attention to our gut then, not do as so many do, and as is well summed up by James Lendall Basford (1845 – 1915):

Men usually take better care of their boots than of their stomachs.

Sparks from the Philosopher's Stone (1882)

Mr James Lendall Basford, a watchmaker and jeweller from Massachusetts, published two books of his own aphorisms — *Sparks from the Philosopher's Stone* in 1882 and *Seven Seventy Seven Sensations* in 1897. He said of these that they were 'the result of ideas which have forced themselves into expression during a period of the author's life, extending from early youth to middle age, amidst the many cares and perplexities of a business life'.[72]

Chapter 26

Fungi and yeasts:
often the early invaders

Why did the Fungus leave the party?
Because there wasn't mushroom
Our job is to make sure that 'Fungus', and his best friend, yeast, do not gate-crash our party!

We are seeing epidemics of chronic fungal infection – so much so that it is almost seen as being normal, but such infections are early signs that the arms race is starting to be lost. Oral thrush in babies is perceived as normal, nappy rash is often fungal and cradle cap is a fungal infection of the scalp. Later in life we see dandruff – a further manifestation of fungal infection. Athlete's foot is a fungal infection of the skin of the feet, especially between the toes – fungi love warm, sweaty areas. Fungal rashes are common and have been given different names to reflect that, like athlete's foot, dhobi itch, jock rot, gym itch, scrot rot, ring worm, tinea, pityriasis and other such. Itching is a symptom characteristic of fungal infection. Various fungi are involved, including candida, *Malassezia furfur*, epidermophyton, microsporum and trichophyton.

The question is, why so many fungal infections? We have a clue – diabetics often present with fungal infections, such as toenail infections where the nail is discoloured and thickened. If blood sugar runs high, sugar oozes onto the skin via sweat and there the fungi get their free lunch and flourish. They also colonise the upper gut in people with carbohydrate-based diets and this results in upper fermenting gut by yeast with all the problems that go with that (Chapter 25). At some point, there is potential for fungi to spill over into the bloodstream and drive inflammatory reactions at faraway sites. We know that gluten will result in a leaky gut in all people – you do not have to be allergic for this to happen. Western diets high in gluten and carbs create a perfect storm for leaky gut, autoimmunity and low-grade infection.

Can we call this infection? I do not care about semantics – the bottom line is that there are many yeast-driven symptoms and pathologies. Many of these are also driven by other microbes because where there are yeasts fermenting, there will also be bacteria doing so because both love to ferment carbohydrates.

My clinical impression is that there are two clear stages to fungal and yeast problems. The first represents the stage where these fungi are growing happily on the sugars which are readily available to them. These infections can be easily dealt with by Groundhog Basic: starve them with the PK diet; kill them with vitamin C; improve the defences with micronutrients, herbs and fungi (as in fungi used in cooking). I do not pretend this is easy, but it is within the powers of us all.

The second stage occurs when fungi are in a 'mycelial' form (from the Greek *'myco'*, fungus, and *'hēlos'*, nail, thereby meaning 'nail of (the) fungus'). Their roots extend across natural barriers of skin and mucous membrane to access sugar directly from our body tissues. Groundhog Basic is an essential starting point, but antifungal drugs will probably be needed in addition.

Table 26.1: Treatment of fungal infections

Location of fungal infection	Treatment – Groundhog Basic plus...
Fungal skin infections	Iodine ointment applied *ad lib*; keep the skin stained yellow Possibly terbinafine 250 mg daily
Fungal nails	Neat Lugol's 12% iodine *ad lib* onto the nails; keep them stained yellow Possibly terbinafine 250 mg daily
Mucous membranes: vagina, perineum, upper airways, bronchi and lungs	Iodine ointment Inhaled iodine in salt pipe (e.g. 4 drops of Lugol's iodine into the salt chamber) for two minutes inhalation four times daily Itraconazole 100 mg daily or fluconazole 50 mg daily. If these are needed for more than one month, then you need blood tests to check your liver function. I recommend such after one, three and six months of treatment. Should abnormalities occur, then they reverse when the drug is stopped, but good micronutrient status is highly protective against any such toxicity
	Lufenuron may be helpful. This drug inhibits chitin synthesis, thereby breaking down fungal cell walls. It is widely used in the veterinary world. Because humans do not have this enzyme system the potential for side effects is minimal
Mucous membranes: gut from mouth to anus	Vitamin C to bowel tolerance Herbal preparations are often very effective. The more herbs you can take and the higher the dose, the better. Many are effective; my favourites are garlic and caprylic acid as coconut oil (in cooking generally and in 'PK *Cordyceps* chocolate' as described in *The PK Cookbook*), and berberine, plant tannins and uva ursi as capsules. Everyone develops their own preferences Pure nystatin powder – this is very effective if you can get it. It is not absorbed into the bloodstream and so high doses, if necessary long term, are very safe An antifungal (or anti-candida) diet does not have to avoid yeast and fungi. Live fungi will be killed in the upper gut by Groundhog Basic. The only reason to avoid them would be because of allergy to them.

Duration of treatment

What most of these drugs do is to prevent the fungus from growing. Time is needed for the fungus to grow out. For infections of mucous membranes, we need several days of treatment; for skin, several weeks; and for nails, several months. A rough rule of thumb (no pun intended!) is that treatment should continue for two months after symptoms have resolved.

> **Linguistic note:** 'Rule of thumb' is often said to derive from a law that allowed a man to beat his wife with a stick as long as it is were no thicker than his thumb. The story goes that in 1782, Judge Sir Francis Buller made this legal ruling. In the following year, James Gillray published a satirical cartoon of Buller, caricaturing him as 'Judge Thumb'. Perhaps Buller has been mis-reported – the phrase was in use before 1782. He was known for being harsh in his punishments, but there is no evidence that he made this ruling. Edward Foss, author of *The Judges of England*, 1870, wrote that, despite investigation, 'no substantial evidence has been found that he ever expressed so ungallant an opinion'. (Craig's note: A little more than ungallant, I would say!)

When you have cleared the fungi, remember not to slip back into old wicked ways or you will simply set up the very conditions that allowed fungi to invade in the first place. Groundhog Basic is for life.

And now, lest you feel cheated, here is the joke you may have been expecting at the start of this chapter:

Why did the mushroom get invited to all the parties?

Because he is a fun-gi!

Part IV

Do you have a chronic infection?
How to diagnose and treat

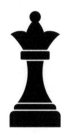

Chapter 27

Chronic infection
Are you infected?

There are literally thousands of microbes with the potential to make themselves at home in our comfortable bodies. Some we know drive pathology, and thankfully we have some near-miraculous diagnostic and therapeutic tools to deal with them. Many chronic infections are well recognised and well treated with prescription antivirals, antibiotics and other antimicrobials. The key to success is to diagnose accurately which microbe is the problem and then decide which antimicrobial, or combination of such, will be effective against that organism. These principles apply to the treatment of all infection.

How do you know if you have a chronic infection?

The symptoms of chronic infection are multiple because:
*   By the time the infections have breached our defences any, and indeed many, organs of the body will be affected. There may be symptoms because of organ inflammation (heat, pain and swelling), organ damage or organ failure.
*   As the body fights infection, this will kick a hole in the energy bucket, so fatigue is an almost universal symptom.

What this means in practical reality is that it is impossible to diagnose the underlying microbes involved with a chronic infection through the clinical picture. The bottom line is that you have to do tests.

It is also the case that once you have one chronic infection, you are likely to have others for the very same reason that you acquired the first (and remember, the common mechanisms of acquiring infection are the four Gs – gobs and guts, genitals and gnats). So, if you suspect you have Lyme disease because of an insect bite (not necessarily a tick), then you are likely also to harbour *Babesia*, *Bartonella* and other such bastards.

However, *'illegitimi non carborundum'* or, 'Don't let the bastards get you down!' (This is a mock Latin idiomatic translation. For purists, perhaps, *'Noli pati a scelestis opprimi'* is closer to the 'real' Latin. In any case, read on!)

Finally, regardless of which infections you are harbouring, the starting point of treatment is always the same – first improve the defences.

At present, we have chronic infections that fall into three artificial groups:

1. **Well-recognised chronic infections that are well dealt with already**: The specifics of treatment of well-recognised chronic infections such as HIV, tuberculosis, hepatitis C and so on are beyond my experience and the scope of this book. However, Groundhog Chronic will greatly improve the response to antimicrobials.

2. **New but less well-recognised chronic infections that are very poorly dealt with – so-called 'stealth infections'**: This is an area in which I have had to become expert because so many of my patients with fatigue are carrying an infectious burden that is making them ill. This includes Lyme (*Borrelia*), *Bartonella*, *Babesia*, *Mycoplasma*, *Chlamydia*, *Rickettsia*, *Yersinia* and others. Chronic fatigue syndrome is my area of clinical expertise and this clinical picture arises when energy delivery mechanisms are impaired. Myalgic encephalitis (ME) is CFS plus inflammation – that is to say, there is an immunological hole, such as chronic infection (but it may be allergy or autoimmunity or all three), in the energy bucket, together with additional symptoms of inflammation. Inflammation is the clinical picture that occurs when the immune system is active, fighting, for example, a chronic infection. (See my book *Diagnosis and Treatment of Chronic Fatigue Syndrome and Myalgic encephalitis – it's mitochondria, not hypochondria!* for much more detail.)

3. **New infections that we have yet to discover:** New diseases are first recognised when patients suffer inexplicable symptoms. The science is often slow to catch

up, so we have a nasty window of time when the conventional doctors deny there is a problem. These doctor 'diagnose' the intellectually risible MUPS (Medically Unexplained Physical Symptoms). There the thinking stops, and the poor patients are handed over to the psychiatrists for Big Pharma strait-jacket, symptom-suppressing drugs. The few practitioners who do believe that their patients are physically ill are denigrated and ostracised by the medical profession and many, like myself, are hounded by the Establishment. Again, see my book *Diagnosis and Treatment of Chronic Fatigue Syndrome and Myalgic Encephalitis* for much more detail – particularly in Chapter 1.

Part of the reason why we are seeing the new epidemics is because the medical profession cannot believe this is possible. It fails to recognise that:

- Our immune systems are declining because of modern diets, pollution (chemical and electromagnetic) and, probably, vaccination
- Climate change means biting insects are moving into new habitats and infecting people who do not have any natural resistance
- We are travelling more than ever before, so infections once confined to one area of the world are now easily spread
- Intensive farming of poultry and pigs offers fresh breeding sites for new microbes to evolve. Since antibiotics are routinely fed to these animals, these new microbes are antibiotic resistant
- Sexually transmitted disease is commonplace
- Doctors, dentists and surgeons may well be unwitting vectors of disease through direct inoculation of virus or prion particles (via vaccination and blood products), hospital environments and procedures.

We have to recognise that we are seeing epidemics of new chronic infections and that conventional doctors are still at the denial stage.

All truth passes through three stages. First, it is ridiculed. Second, it is violently opposed. Third, it is accepted as being self-evident.
Arthur Schopenhauer, German philosopher (1788 – 1860)

I am at the start of this journey and on a very steep learning curve. However, already it is very clear to me that the best results are achieved by patients learning about their illness and fashioning their own recovery. What follows are the Rules of the Game and the Tools of the Trade to allow them to progress. It is like playing cricket – we all use the same rules and tools, but each player evolves a distinct and unique style which additionally relies on physique, talent, character, timing and very many other variables, all of which affect the outcome.

If, despite Groundhog Acute, there continue to be persistent symptoms of inflammation, that may point to a nasty infection that has become entrenched and is resistant to Groundhog alone. In this case, we need modern weapons of warfare – Exocet missiles and atomic bombs. Prescription antimicrobials may be essential to get ahead in the arms race. Antibiotics, antivirals and antifungals have specific rather than general actions, so we need to do our best to identify our enemy. Good diagnosis will require good tests.

The word 'diagnosis' stems from the Ancient Greek διάγνωσις (diágnōsis), which in turn derives from διά (diá, 'apart') plus γιγνώσκειν (gignóskein, 'to learn'). You will see from what follows that this is a good description – patients must *learn* about their symptoms and signs of illness and about the tests available and use this information to tease *apart* which chronic infection(s) may be the culprit from the many possibilities that could be at play.

However, Groundhog Chronic will greatly enhance the efficacy of antimicrobials and substantially reduce the chance of side effects and complications.

Groundhog interventions are essentially defensive protocols, but remember that the Spartans not only used their shields to defend themselves but also as a weapon with which to beat their enemies to death! Do not forget or lose your shield.

Spartan mothers knew this and had this advice for their sons going off to battle:

Come back with your shield, or on it.
        Plutarch, *Moralia, 241* Greek-Roman biographer (AD 46 – AD 120)

Chapter 28

Principles of diagnosis of chronic 'stealth' infections
Which tests?

There may be clues from the clinical picture (see below), but definite diagnosis will require laboratory tests. These are expensive, but we can increase the chances of a positive diagnosis by first considering symptoms and signs. A vital and powerful symptom of a chronic stealth infection is failure to respond to Groundhog interventions. Regardless of whether you do or do not test positive for a chronic stealth infection, Groundhog must be in place for long-term good health, especially for old crones like me – so just do it and do it now. Indeed, I know that many of my patients must have been cured through Groundhog alone. I say that because these stealth infections are common, so many of my patients who have recovered must, unknowingly, have suffered from them.

Symptoms and signs of chronic infection

History
The clinical history is perhaps the most important tool for diagnosis. Start when the symptoms began – which may be decades earlier. The list below is not comprehensive, but put in order of probability based on my clinical experience.

Table 28.1: Assessing the history of chronic infection

How the symptoms started	Possible diagnosis	Useful tests to support diagnosis in order of priority
Sudden 'flu-like illness, fever, malaise. Feeling ghastly: • Unable to do anything, let alone work • Bedbound for some days • Perhaps swollen glands in neck, armpits, groin • Perhaps went a bit yellow • Perhaps pericarditis and chest pain • At the time blood tests may have been 'a bit wrong but nothing to worry about'	Human herpes virus 4 (HHV4) or 'Epstein Barr virus' which causes glandular fever	Armin laboratory tests: • Elispot • IgG antibody titre • IgM antibody titre • DNA by PCR. These tests are available from www.naturalhealthworldwide.com. A raised IgG is typically interpreted as evidence of past exposure, *ergo* no treatment necessary as not active. However, it does not exclude the possibility that a microbe is driving pathology
Ditto	Human herpes virus 6 (HHV6) or 'roseola'	IgG/IgM antibodies DNA PCR
Ditto	Coxsackie virus	IgG/IgA antibodies
Ditto	Human herpes virus 5 (HHV5) Cytomegalovirus (CMV)	Elispot
As above with localising signs, e.g. shingles, chickenpox (Cold sores and genital herpes are also herpes viruses but rarely trigger CFS/ME)	Other herpes viruses. All herpes viruses target the brain and immune system. Once in the body all herpes viruses persist for life	Elispot for *Varicella zoster* (shingles, chicken pox) Elispot for HHV1 and HHV2 IgG antibody titre
Vaccination – I estimate that one in 10 of my CFS/ME patients have their disease triggered or worsened by vaccination	These are designed to switch on the immune system, with the potential to trigger autoimmunity and allergy	There may be positive IgG titres to virus

Vaccination	We know some retroviruses have been present in vaccination such as SV 40 (simian vacuolating virus 40, or simian virus 40, a polyomavirus that is found in both monkeys and humans). The jury is still out with respect to XMRV (xenotropic murine leukaemia virus-related virus – see historical note).	It is almost impossible to get retroviral tests done
Acute gastroenteritis (or indeed any gut symptom such as pain, bloating, reflux, diarrhoea, constipation, abnormally formed stools)	Fermenting gut Inflammatory bowel disease Mycobacterium avium subspecies paratuberculosis (MAP) Parasite or unfriendly gut microbes e.g. *H pylori*, *Giardia*, amoebiasis blastocystis hominis	Comprehensive digestive stool analysis e.g. Doctors Data or Genova I know of no commercial test for MAP Other tests are available from www.naturalhealthworldwide.com
Possibly a tick bite and bull's eye rash but probably none such. As with *Borrelia*, *Babesia* and *Bartonella*, any insect bite could transmit many infections Possibly rash and arthritic condition Often no clear onset	Lyme disease – *Borrelia burgdorferi*, *Borrelia myamotoi*	Armin labs: Elispot Seraspot (Often antibody tests are negative – this does not exclude the diagnosis). Tests are available from www.naturalhealthworldwide.com
As with *Borrelia*, could be acquired through insect bites. Virtually all mammals harbour *Bartonella*. *Bartonella* classically follows a cat scratch, but absence of such does not exclude the diagnosis	*Bartonella* – may cause a PUO (pyrexia – fever (FUO) – of unknown origin)	Armin: Elispot IgG/IgM antibodies DNA PCR (polymerase chain reaction) Tests are available from www.naturalhealthworldwide.com
Insect bites	*Babesia* – may cause a PUO	Armin: Elispot IgG/IgM antibodies *Babesia* DNA PCR Tests are available from www.naturalhealthworldwide.com

How the symptoms started	Possible diagnosis	Useful tests to support diagnosis in order of priority
Insect bites	*Rickettsia*	Elispot *Ehrlichia* Elispot *Anaplasma*
Ditto	*Yersinia*	Elispot *Yersinia*
Chest infection or pneumonia (may be atypical 'walking pneumonia' – that is, the patient is not very ill). I seem to be seeing many new cases – at least four in 2017	*Mycoplasma pneumoniae*	IgG antibodies
Ditto	*Chlamydia pneumoniae*	Elispot IgG antibodies Tests are available from www.naturalhealthworldwide.com
Sexually transmitted disease	*Chlamydia trachomatis* HIV, Hepatitis C, syphilis, herpes, HPV, gonorrhoea, trichomonas, bacterial vaginosis	Get screening tests at a Special Clinic Elispot IgG antibodies
Recurrent chest, upper respiratory or sinus infections	Chronic septic focus, e.g. bronchiectasis	Chest X-ray Sputum sample (but often false negative) *Aspergillus* precipitin test IgG IgM and IgA antibodies
Joint pains and arthritis	Inflammation driven by allergy to microbes from the fermenting gut OR Allergy to a virus – so-called 'reactive arthritis'	No direct tests Auto-antibody studies may help Investigations for the fermenting gut: comprehensive digestive stool analysis, e.g. Doctors Data or Genova. Tests are available from www.naturalhealthworldwide.com

Historical note: Judy A Mikovits PHD is an ME/CFS researcher and was previously the research director at the Whittemore Peterson Institute (WPI – now the Nevada Center for Biomedical Research). Dr Mikovits led the team that published a paper suggesting a connection between the XMRV (xenotropic murine leukaemia virus-related virus) retrovirus and ME/CFS; it was thought that one possible route of transmission was vaccinations. As a result of this paper, Mikovits felt the full force of scientific prejudices regarding ME/CFS, and eventually she was fired from the WPI in 2011. After her sacking, there was a legal dispute with the WPI – Dr Mikovits was actually arrested at this time. All charges, including criminal charges of theft, brought by the WPI against Dr Mikovits were eventually dropped. This book is not the place for a full recounting of the circumstances surrounding these events but, for example, at one time, Dr Mikovits was banned from even setting foot on the NCI (National Cancer Institute) campus, a prohibition which would be enforced by security. The full story is told in the excellent book *Plague: One Scientist's Intrepid Search for the Truth About Human Retroviruses and Chronic Fatigue Syndrome (ME/CFS), Autism and Other Diseases*, written by Kent Heckenlively (a former attorney) and Judy Mikovits.

Current symptoms and signs

Chronic infections often start with local symptoms of inflammation, such as sore throat, head cold, chest infection, gastroenteritis or urinary tract infection, but as the microbe makes itself comfortably at home in your body, the symptoms then become more general and, indeed, may start to trigger pathology (disease symptoms). Many chronic so-called 'degenerative' conditions we know are driven by infection. This includes most cases of dementia (herpes viruses, Lyme) and Parkinson's (Lyme) and many cases of autoimmunity, cancer, arterial disease, arthritis and, of course, CFS/ME. Indeed, with any inflammatory pathology, always think and look for an infectious cause.

When I was at medical school I learned that syphilis was the 'great mimic' because it can cause almost any pathology. Syphilis had to be thought of in almost every differential diagnosis (list of possible diagnoses to consider). Lyme too is caused by a spirochete (a specialised type of bacteria) with similar potential for damage and mimicry. This case report demonstrates the possibility for mimicry:

> ***Lyme disease-induced polyradiculopathy mimicking amyotrophic lateral sclerosis (ALS)****: (ALS is a form of motor neurone disease.) 'The initial electrodiagnostic test showed widespread active and chronic denervation findings. The initial physical and electrodiagnostic findings were suggestive of Amyotrophic Lateral Sclerosis (ALS). However, blood serology indicated possible Lyme disease. Thus, the patient was treated with doxycycline.* The clinical and electrodiagnostic findings were resolved with the treatment.'[73]*

Interpretation of tests

No test is perfect. All must be interpreted in the light of the particular patient's history, and all patients are unique. This is what makes medicine an art as much as a science. So much modern Western medicine has been condensed to simple algorithms based on a drug end-result so that real pathology is missed. Patients suffer and die needlessly. Nowhere is this a greater issue than in the interpretation of tests. Any result is taken as absolute. So often I see patients who have been told that all their test results are normal and that they must therefore either not be ill or are hypochondriacs. Nowhere is this worse than in the field of CFS/ME.

There are several possible mechanisms that form the basis of tests to decide if chronic infection is present:

- A false negative result means: this does not exclude infection
- A false positive result means: there may be, or has been, microbe exposure but it is no longer a clinical problem.

You may need different tests for different microbes, depending on where it is living in the body and whether the immune system is fighting it with antibodies or with white-cell foot soldiers.

---

*See also Chapter 33 where I discuss the use of doxycycline in the treatment of Lyme disease.

Table 28.2: Interpreting test results

Test	Mechanism	Notes
Can that microbe be seen or grown in tissue culture?	Not all can be Viruses cannot be grown in culture	False negative results are common. A positive result makes it very likely you are harbouring that microbe.
PCR (polymerase chain reaction)?	If positive, then that microbe is present	But false negatives abound. You will only get a positive result if the microbe you are looking for is present in the tissue sample that has been taken
Are there IgM antibodies to that microbe?	This is part of the acute immune response	If positive, then the immune system is fighting that microbe BUT False negatives abound with stealth infections
Are there IgG antibodies to that microbe?	This forms part of immune memory	We commonly see a positive result which may well mean all is well – i.e. that microbe has been dealt with and kicked into touch by the immune system
		However, sometimes there are very high IgG responses which may suggest the immune system is still fighting a battle*
Are there IgA antibodies to that microbe?	Tests only apply to microbes living on mucous membranes, such as *Mycoplasma pneumoniae*	False negatives possible
Elispot testing looks at how the white T-cell soldiers are reacting with cytokines to a particular microbe. (This is also known as the 'lymphocyte transformation test' because the normally quiet white-cell soldiers transform into fighting lunatics)	This test is very sensitive, specific and clinically relevant	A positive result means the immune system is fighting the particular infection being tested for. This is a very good test for infection with: • a high level of sensitivity (i.e. false negatives are uncommon) and • a high level of specificity (i.e. it is the microbe you are looking at and not another)

Test	Mechanism	Notes
White cell counts	May be high during acute infection	Help these with Groundhog Acute
	May be low with chronic infection…	… as the immune system becomes exhausted because it is running out of raw materials or energy. Treat this with Groundhog Chronic

*Table Footnote: For example, finding a high IgG antibody titre is generally thought to be simply evidence of past infection. However, we know that all herpes viruses persist in the body for life, so if they have been there in the past they will be present today. Once comfortably installed in the body, they have the potential to drive many other nasty diseases (see Chapter 2). Their targeting of the brain and immune system explains many symptoms. I suspect it is this group of viruses that are responsible for many cases of post-viral CFS/ME. Dr Martin Lerner showed that EBV (Epstein Barr virus, also known as HHV4, 'mono' and glandular fever) was causally involved in 81% of cases of post-viral CFS. (See Appendix 6 of our book *Diagnosis and Treatment of Chronic Fatigue Syndrome and Myalgic Encephalitis – it's mitochondria, not hypochondria* for much more detail on this.)

A general rule of thumb amongst clinicians is that if the 'antibody titre' is five times higher than baseline, then consider pursuing an antiviral strategy. What is so interesting is that Dr Lerner showed that the antiviral titre (EBV nuclear antigen and EBV viral capsid antigen) fell with effective treatment and that this was paralleled by clinical improvement. This allows an objective measure of progress. Armin laboratories now offer Elispot testing for EBV, and this is a very useful tool. Again, as the immune system defeats the virus, the level of positivity comes down – this is a very helpful clinical tool.

How to get help

It has taken me decades to realise that I cannot help all the sick people in the world. With Craig's help, together with the wonderful team of Dan Grey, Kathryn Twinn and Carolyn May, we have set up a website that allows any patient to contact any doctor, qualified health practitioner or experienced patient, and consult on any symptom or method of treatment (www.naturalhealthworldwide.com). We are using this as a training system for practitioners. The idea is that there are many frontline 'registrar' practitioners who can teach Groundhog. Done well this alone will cure many patients. However, should they get stuck, registrars can consult with, or refer to, a second-line 'consultant' practitioner, such as myself or other experienced doctors, for a trouble-shooting session.

Summary

Diagnosis depends on:
- A high level of clinical suspicion – if you don't look you don't see!
- Good tests and interpretation of these – in this respect, diagnostic tests are essential.
- Response to treatment: All diagnosis is hypothesis, which must then be put to the test. However, always remember this may not be the sole cause of symptoms.

Finally, once one infection has become established, one must recognise that other microbes are more likely to get into the body, perhaps for the same reasons that the first microbes got in – that is, poor defences. So, the existence of one microbe may indicate that other, as yet unidentified, microbes may also be present. The point here is that it will never be sufficient just to target a particular microbe that has been identified. Improving the defences is as vital a part of attacking microbes as is targeting particular microbes. Having had one debilitating infection, always return to Groundhog Chronic. You will find Craig and me there too!

Finally, I stress once again, these chronic infections *do* exist and that tackling them can be the key to recovery for many patients.

A famous European philosopher sums up where we are at this moment:

There are two ways to be fooled. One is to believe what isn't true; the other is to refuse to believe what is true.

Søren Kierkegaard, Danish philosopher (1813 – 1855)

Do not be fooled either way!

Chapter 29

The general principles of treating stealth infection

Remember it is a numbers game. You have symptoms because that microbe has overwhelmed your defences. Your immune system, your standing army, is fighting and that battle ground is adding to your symptoms because it is a battleground of inflammation. You must do anything and everything you can to reduce the infectious load and the friendly fire that results from the battle scene.

Improve the defences

Start with Groundhog Acute. The bowel tolerance method for vitamin C (page 57) is especially helpful because bowel tolerance is also a measure of your infectious load. It is very heartening to know that you are winning the battle because your bowel tolerance should fall in parallel with the infection.

When that has been achieved, move on to Groundhog Chronic.

Antimicrobials

Use whatever antimicrobials are available that target the microbe concerned. For details of regimes, read on in the chapters that follow. The treatments may well sound aggressive to you, and many of my patients are bitterly opposed to antibiotics often for good reason (perhaps because they have been employed without Groundhog), but remember, all these infections drive nasty pathologies – you do not get ill because you get old, you get ill because you are infected! Infections kill.

What to expect

You may worsen initially. As you start treatment you may see a temporary worsening of symptoms. I think there are two possible reasons for this – namely, Herxheimer reactions, and detoxing. Both are good signs but miserable and uncomfortable.

• A Herxheimer reaction is an allergic reaction to microbial body parts as the antimicrobial kills. Yippee – this means microbes must be dead!
• A detox reaction is a short-term poisoning as toxins, such as bacterial endotoxin, are released systemically. Yippee – this means one is reducing one's toxic load!

However, many patients are already so ill they cannot afford to be made worse. In this event one must just reduce the level of treatment until the reactions have reduced to a tolerable level, then build up again. Again, for these reasons, I suggest starting with Groundhog Acute, establish Groundhog Chronic so the patient is feeling reasonably comfortable, then add in the herbal and prescription Exocet missiles and atomic bombs as described in the chapters that follow.

Duration of treatment

When treatment is effective, the numbers of microbes fall exponentially. You will get to a stage when symptoms resolve but microbes will still be present. Do not stop treatment but you can reduce the intensity so long as the symptoms do not return. (Absence of symptoms tells us microbe numbers are low.) A rule of thumb for treating chronic infections with antibiotics is to continue for two months after symptoms have resolved. However, Groundhog Chronic should be continued for life – that is, if, like me, you are aiming to live to 120.

Note from Craig – Perhaps it is time to pay the bookies a visit, Sarah? Last year a 60-year-old female placed a £100 bet at odds of 2000-1 that she should reach 120 years of age. Think of the party we could have with £200,000 or so! Well, depending on inflation rates in the next few decades anyway.

Chapter 30

Groundhog Chronic

As we age, we acquire infections. Fifteen per cent of my DNA is comprised of retro virus. So is yours. I was inoculated with Salk polio vaccine between 1957 and 1966, so I will probably have simian virus 40 (SV 40), a known carcinogen. I am probably carrying the chickenpox, measles, mumps and rubella viruses because I suffered those as a child. I was also a bit spotty, so *Proprionibacterium acnes* may be a potential problem. At least 90% of us have been infected with Epstein Barr virus. I have been bitten by insects and ticks from all over the British Isles so I could also be carrying Lyme (*Borrelia*), *Bartonella*, *Babesia* and perhaps others. I have been a cat owner and could well test positive for *Bartonella*. I have suffered several fractures which have healed, but I know within that scar tissue will be lurking some microbes – feed them some sugar and they will multiply and give me arthritis. I have had dental abscesses in the past and have one root filling which undoubtedly will also harbour microbes. In the past, I have consumed a high-carb diet which inevitably results in a fermenting gut. On the good side, my puritanical upbringing means I have been free from STDs (thank you, Mum).

As you have read, we now know all these microbes have the potential to drive nasty diseases, such as leukaemia, lymphoma, other cancers, dementia, Parkinson's, heart disease, autoimmunity and so on. I cannot eliminate them from my body; I have to live with them. I too am part of the arms race. Of course, this is a race I will (eventually) lose, but I will settle for losing it when I am 120. I am hoping that Groundhog Chronic will handicap my assailants and stack the odds in my favour.

So, as we age and/or acquire stealth infections, we all need Groundhog Chronic. It is an extension of Groundhog Basic. Most people will end up doing something between the two, according to their health and history, but as you get older you have to work harder to stay well.

Youth is wasted on the young.

Oscar Wilde (1854 – 1900)

Table 30.1: Groundhog Chronic

What to do	Why	What I do My patients always ask me what I do. I am no paragon of virtue, but I may have to become one eventually
The paleo-ketogenic diet: • high fat and fibre • very low carb • probiotic foods like kefir and sauerkraut • no dairy or grains • just two meals a day and no snacking Source the best quality foods you can find and afford – organic is a great start	See our books *Prevent and Cure Diabetes – delicious diets not dangerous drugs* for the 'Why' and *The PK Cookbook – go paleo-ketogenic and get the best of both worlds* for the 'How'	Yes, I do the PK diet 95% of the time. I do allow myself a glass of cider at weekends Other liberties if eating out or socialising, but my friends are all becoming PK-adapted too!
Eat daily food within a 10-hour window of time…	…so there are 14 hours a day when your stomach is empty; this keeps it acid and so decreases the chances of microbes invading. It also maintains ketosis	Nearly there… breakfast at 8 am and supper at 6.30 pm
Consider episodic fasting one day a week	This gives the gut a lovely rest and a chance to heal and repair	I do this some weeks. The trouble is I am greedy and love food
A basic package of nutritional supplements – multi-vitamins, multi-minerals and vitamin D	A good multivitamin and Sunshine salt 1 teaspoon daily with food A dessertspoon of hemp oil	Yes, I do this

What to do	Why	What I do My patients always ask me what I do. I am no paragon of virtue, but I may have to become one eventually
Glutathione 250 mg daily Iodine 25 mg weekly	We live in such a toxic world we are inevitably exposed to poisons. Glutathione and iodine are helpful detox molecules (Note that some people cannot tolerate iodine in high doses)	Yes, I do this
Vitamin C to 90% of bowel tolerance, including 5 grams last thing at night. Remember your personal tolerance will change with age, diet and circumstances	With age, influenza becomes a major killer. With Groundhog Chronic you need never even get it	Yes, I currently need 8 grams in 24 hours but I never get colds or influenza
Lugol's iodine 12% 2 drops daily in water	Swill this around your mouth and swallow last thing at night	Yes, I do this
Make sure your First Aid box is stocked (see page 215)…	…so, you have all your ammo to hand to hit new symptoms hard and fast	Yes, even when I go away I take this – often to treat sickly others
Sleep 8-9 hours between 10 pm and 7 am Regular 'power nap' in the day	More in winter, less in summer Good sleep is as vital as a good diet	Yes, I do this
Exercise within limits. By this I mean you should feel fully recovered next day If well enough, once a week push those limits, so you get your pulse up to 120 beats per min and all your muscles ache It is never too late to start!	No pain, no gain Muscle loss is part of ageing – exercise slows this right down It also helps to physically dislodge microbes from their hiding places. (I suspect massage works similarly)	Yes, thankfully I am one of those who can and do enjoy exercise
Take supplements for the raw materials for connective tissue, such as glucosamine. Bone broth is the best!	With age we become less good at healing and repair	Yes, I do this

Herbs, spices and fungi in cooking	Use your favourite herbs, spices and fungi in cooking and food, and lots of them	Yes – I love food!
Consider herbs to improve the defences (see Chapter 13)	*Astragalus, Cordyceps* and rhodiola	Sometimes, when they are in stock and I remember
Address energy delivery mechanisms, as below	See our book *Diagnosis and Treatment of Chronic Fatigue Syndrome and Myalgic Encephalitis: it's mitochondria, not hypochondria*	Yes, Craig – I've got the book!
Take the mitochondrial package of supplements daily, vis: • co-enzyme Q10, 100 grams • niacinamide slow-release 1500 mg • acetyl L-carnitine 500 mg • D-ribose 5-10 grams at night if you have really overdone things	With age, fatigue becomes an increasing issue because our mitochondrial engines start to slow. The ageing process is determined by mitochondria. Look after them	Yes, but I don't take carnitine because I eat meat and my digestion is good
Mitochondria may be going slow because of toxins so consider tests of toxic load to see if you need to do any detox	A good all-rounder is Genova urine screen with DMSA, 15 mg per kg of body weight. You can get this test through https://naturalhealthworldwide.com/	I have not got around to doing this but I know I should
Check your living space for electromagnetic pollution	You can hire a detection meter from www.healthy-house.co.uk/electro/meters-and-monitors	Yes, the cordless phone has gone I never hold a mobile phone to my ear – I use the speaker Turn wifi off at night

What to do	Why	What I do
		My patients always ask me what I do. I am no paragon of virtue, but I may have to become one eventually
Review any prescription medication – all drugs are potential toxins. The need for drugs is likely to be symptomatic of failure to apply Groundhog	Ask yourself, why are you taking drugs? See our book *Sustainable Medicine*. Once Groundhog Chronic is in place, many drugs can be stopped. Taking prescription drugs is the fourth commonest cause of death in Westerners	I never take symptom-suppressing medication. This has allowed full and now pain-free recovery from three broken necks (horses again)
Consider tests of adrenal and thyroid function since these glands fatigue with age and chronic infection	Thyroid bloods tests and adrenal saliva tests available through https://naturalhealthworldwide.com/ Core temperatures are helpful for fine-tuning adrenal and thyroid function with glandular – see 'CFS: conducting the orchestra' at www.drmyhill.co.uk/wiki/ Conducting_the_CFS_orchestra_–_how_to_put_yourself_in_charge	I find glandulars very helpful and currently take thyroid glandular 60 mg in the morning and 30 mg at midday plus adrenal glandular 250 mg twice daily
Heat and light	Always keep warm Sunbathe at every opportunity Holidays in warm climates with sunbathing and swimming are excellent for killing infections and detoxing Do not forget that hyperthermia and light together are a good treatment for chronic infections (see Chapter 11)	I am a pyromaniac – my kitchen is lovely and warm with a wood-fired range. I work in my conservatory with natural light. I sunbathe as often as wet Wales permits
Use your brain	Foresight: Avoid risky actions like kissing and unprotected sex Caution: Avoid vaccinations; choose travel destinations with care Circumspection: Do not suppress symptoms with drugs; treat breaches of the skin seriously	I have to say that with age this is much less of an issue – no vaccinations; no foreign travel except to the Continent to see my daughter and to give lectures

Once again, remember, as Oscar Wilde said, though perhaps for different reasons than the risk of infection:

A kiss may ruin a human life
> Oscar Wilde in *A Woman of No Importance* (Is there ever such a thing? Craig)
> (16 October 1854 – 30 November 1900)

If you are tiring from Groundhog, be inspired by these quotes:

We are what we repeatedly do. Excellence, then, is not an act, but a habit.
> Idiomatic translation by Will Durrant in *The Story of Philosophy*
> of the original quotation by Aristotle, which read,

Excellence is an art won by training and habituation.
> Aristotle (384 BC – 322 BC)

repetitio est mater studiorum – *'repetition is the mother of all learning'*
> Old Latin Proverb

consuetudinis magna vis est – *'the force of habit is great'*
Cicero (106 BC – 43 BC, assassinated for his opposition to Mark Antony, Cicero's last words were purportedly, 'There is nothing proper about what you are doing, soldier, but do try to kill me properly'.)

Chapter 31

Chronic infection of the gut:
microbes that have moved in and made themselves at home in the gut wall

Chronic infection of the gut comes about as a result of microbes which have moved in and made themselves at home in the gut wall. The commonest I see in clinical practice are the parasites. I always consider the possibility of parasites where there are any gut symptoms. This is such an important diagnosis to make because it is relatively easy to treat with good results. Diagnosis can be made with a comprehensive digestive stool analysis including a request for parasites. You can order this test through https://naturalhealthworldwide.com/lab_tests.php You will also need Elispot to pick up *Yersinia*.

Once a parasite has become established you may need medication over and above Groundhog Acute (page 110) to get rid of it.

Table 31.1: Treating parasites with prescription drugs

Parasite	Treatment	Comments
Amoebiasis – *Dientamoeba fragilis* and *Entamoeba histolytica*	Metronidazole 400 mg three times daily for two weeks	This works reliably well. I have not seen success with herbals. Protect the microbiome (see Chapters 8 and 37)
Giardia lamblia	Ditto	Ditto

Parasite	Treatment	Comments
Blastocystis hominis	Metronidazole does not work. I have one patient who cleared this with Groundhog Acute. Otherwise one needs doxycycline 100 mg twice daily and paromomycin 500 mg three times daily for two weeks	This is a real pig of a parasite to get rid of. The experiences of other practitioners can be seen at www.badbugs.org Protect the microbiome – see Chapters 8 and 37
Cryptosporidia	Good chance of getting rid of this with Groundhog Basic – that is, vitamin C to bowel tolerance (see Chapter 9). Azithromycin 500 mg daily for five days	Protect the microbiome – see Chapters 8 and 37
Roundworm, hookworm, whipworm, threadworm and pinworm	Mebendazole 100 mg: one dose works reliably well – a very safe drug	Threadworm is a very common problem in children. Where there is a problem, treat the whole family. No impact on the microbiome

Linguistic note: Derivation of 'parasite' – from the Latin, *parasitus*, and Greek, *parasitos*, meaning 'feeding beside', from para (besides, beyond) and sit(os), (grain, food). In Ancient Greek, this word was applied to a person who received free meals from a host in return for amusing, sometimes even impudent, conversation at the dinner table, or indeed often the 'cost' of the meal was blatant flattery bestowed upon the host. The parasites that are the topic of this chapter give nothing in return!

Ulcerative colitis

This occurs when the microbiome of the large intestine becomes abnormal and the microbes invade the gut wall to drive chronic inflammation. This too is another manifestation of the fermenting gut, and faecal bacteriotherapy (page 232) has been a really successful treatment. Importantly, this treatment may result in a complete cure. I have seen several patients greatly improve simply with Groundhog Acute followed by Groundhog Chronic.

Helicobacter pylori

This is a common cause of gut symptoms and should be routinely tested for where these are inexplicable. The diagnosis can only be made by tests. The most convenient is a breath test available from https://naturalhealthworldwide.com/lab_tests.php. A breath test is best because, if positive, it tells you there is current infection. This means you can retest after treatment to make sure it has worked. Chronic *H. pylori* is a risk factor for cancer and heart disease.

One study showed a 30% cure rate with four weeks of just 5 grams of vitamin C daily.[74] This suggests to me that Groundhog Acute is highly likely to be effective. One can at least try and retest to confirm. If this fails, then antibiotics are needed, such as amoxicillin 1 gram and clarithromycin 500 mg, both twice daily for one week with a proton pump inhibitor.

Diverticulitis

Diverticulitis is an inevitable result of Western diets. Little pockets form in the large bowel which can become acutely inflamed, producing symptoms of a left-sided appendicitis. Treatment of an acute infection must always be taken seriously because there is a risk of rupture with peritonitis. Put in place Groundhog Acute but also, I suggest, doxycycline 100 mg twice daily and continued for at least two days after symptoms have settled. Groundhog Chronic prevents recurrence.

Crohn's disease

Crohn's disease is named after Burrill Bernard Crohn (13 June 1884 – 29 July 1983), an American gastroenterologist, who decided to become a doctor so that he could help his father with his terrible indigestion. Crohn was also a painter of note (in watercolours) and a scholar of the US Civil War. He practised medicine until he was 90 years old.

The cause of Crohn's is uncertain but research has shown the presence of a tuberculosis-like organism called *Mycobacterium avium*, subspecies para-tuberculosis, present in the gut of Crohn's patients.[75] Crohn's may also be caused by *Yersinia enterocolitica* – see below.

Antibiotics are used in some centres to eradicate this and cure Crohn's. This approach is not widely available – the drugs are expensive and must be given long term, which can be up two years and beyond according to the study above. In the few patients I have treated, Groundhog Acute has been highly effective.

This list of potential enemies may seem overwhelming, but remember that Groundhog Acute will do you for most of them. However, if not, then we do have the antibiotics ready to come to our aid.

Yersinia enterocolitis

Yersinia may present with an acute gastroenteritis, but then chronic symptoms persist. This infection is often overlooked. Again, if not diagnosed and treated, the infection will become entrenched in the gut wall causing chronic gut symptoms. It may spread to other areas, causing arthritis and eye, skin and renal disease. *Yersina pestis* was transmitted by rat fleas and caused the Black Death or Plague. Now we have *Yersinia enterocolitica*, which infects the gut with TB-like lesions. Always think of this microbe in anyone with Crohn's disease.

Diagnosis requires a high index of suspicion. It may appear in a stool sample or antibody test, but Elispot test is the most reliable.

Treatment

- Groundhog Chronic
- Antibiotics: doxycycline 100 grams twice daily, possibly ciproxin.[76]

Chapter 32

Epstein Barr virus (EBV) and other herpes viruses

If you have skipped straight to this page, then I reiterate: first improve the defences. So, you must use Groundhog Acute moving on to Groundhog Chronic. My policy is to hit the microbes as hard as you can with all the ammo that you can muster at one fell swoop. I say this because, all too often, I see patients who have been treated for chronic EBV infection but only received the antiviral of choice, and this has failed. When this has happened, where do you go from there?

EBV, glandular fever or 'mono'

We know this is the commonest trigger of post-viral chronic fatigue syndrome (CFS) because of the work of Dr Martin Lerner. He showed that in 81% of cases, EBV was causal. Looked at the other way around, it has been estimated that an acute fatigue syndrome (4-16 weeks) follows in 47% of cases of glandular fever. Altogether, 9-22% of cases of glandular fever will progress to CFS. These statistics alone make glandular fever a serious illness which should be treated aggressively. Do look here – www.treatmentcenterforcfs.com – for full details of Dr Lerner's work and links to all his professional and CFS publications and papers – 204 in total, of which 18 directly address CFS/ME. Also, please see Appendix 6 of my book *Diagnosis and Treatment of CFS/ME – it's mitochondria, not hypochondria* for much more detail on Dr Lerner's many studies on valaciclovir, valganciclovir and EBV.

Indeed, EBV has been associated with cancer, dementia and at least 33 types of autoimmunity, including multiple sclerosis and rheumatoid arthritis – it really is a very nasty virus. See the following studies that demonstrate just how nasty EBV can be:

1. Epstein-Barr virus in systemic autoimmune diseases– by Draborg et al.[77] This review focuses on systemic lupus erythematosus (SLE), rheumatoid arthritis (RA) and Sjögren's syndrome (SS).
2. Epstein-Barr virus: its connection to a host of different diseases – by Barker.[78] This article looks at cancer and autoimmune diseases and references 34 articles.
3. The role of Epstein-Barr virus infection in the development of autoimmune thyroid diseases – by Janegova et al.[79]
4. Epstein-Barr virus in multiple sclerosis by Bagert.[80]
5. The epidemiology of EBV and its association with malignant disease (chapter 53 in *Human Herpes Viruses: Biology, Therapy, and Immunoprophylaxis* by Hjalgrim et al.[81]

Diagnosis

Any post-viral syndrome that has been triggered by glandular fever makes it likely that EBV is causing ongoing immune activation which in turn causes widespread inflammation and kicks a hole in the energy bucket. Blood tests for IgG and IgM antibodies are a good start because they will tell you if the immune system has ever met EBV. If IgM is high, then that suggests there is current infection and so antiviral treatment should start. Hitherto, a rule of thumb has been to start antiviral treatment if the IgG antibody level is five times higher than baseline. However, Armin laboratories now have Elispot tests for EBV and that is likely to be more accurate. Tests are available through https://naturalhealthworldwide.com/. If these are positive, start antivirals as below, both prescription and herbal.

Treatment

Chinese skullcap (Scutellaria baicalensis)

Stephen Buhner, a widely respected medical herbalist, advocates Chinese skullcap for treating EBV. This does seem to be a remarkably safe herb. It kills viruses in many ways, from inhibiting neuraminidase and haemaglutinin production, viral replication and viral entry into host cells, to reducing cytokine cascades and being directly toxic to viruses. He recommends using the root as a powder, 1-3 grams taken three times daily. As with treating many infections, one can suffer Herxheimer (microbe die-off) effects (see page 232).[82]

Other herbs for EBV

Buhner advocates many other herbs for EBV and herpes viruses generally. I would recommend any on the basis of price and availability. High on my list would come:

- oxymatrine
- neem and
- artemesia.

Valaciclovir

In a study of 106 patients with EBV-triggered CFS/ME, Lerner has shown valaciclovir to be effective.[83] Where patients had other herpes viruses, such as HHV5 and HHV6, he added in valganciclovir. I am not a fan of the latter because it is expensive and toxic. I would recommend using valaciclovir in conjunction with herbal preparations in order to enhance its efficacy. (See Chapter 13 for how to enhance the efficacy with herbals – namely, make sure you are using *Astragalus*, rhodiola and *Cordyceps*.)

Practical details – prescription antivirals

Lerner prescribed valaciclovir at a dose rate of 1 gram every six hours (that is, 4 grams per day). For heavier patients, the dose was 1.5 grams every six hours and for lighter patients correspondingly less. A Herxheimer response, with worsening of symptoms and 'energy score' (as measured by the validated Energy Index Point Score® (EIPS®)) continuing for two to six weeks after treatment began was a good prognostic omen. Increasing energy score and decreasing symptoms were apparent at the fifth to sixth month of continuing valaciclovir. As the drug was continued, clinical energy scores were substantially improved and more normal life restored. These clinical improvements were accompanied by improvement in ECG monitoring.

As improvement occurred, the valaciclovir dose was then decreased to 1 gram two times a day, continued for six to 12 weeks, and then stopped. A rough rule of thumb is that treatment should be continued for at least two months after clinical symptoms have resolved. However, I have two patients who did not start to improve until one year of treatment. Lerner stated that approximately 20% of EBV-triggered CFS patients required maintenance valaciclovir to prevent clinical relapse. However, my guess is that with Groundhog Chronic this figure would reduce.

Valaciclovir does appear to be a remarkably safe drug. There is potential for kidney toxicity, so it is wise to monitor creatinine levels at the start of treatment, then at one, three and six months. However, my experience is that doing Groundhog Chronic will greatly reduce the possibility of kidney toxicity.

I have known for years that a particularly helpful treatment for my CFS patients is magnesium, by either mouth or injection. This is an essential mineral for good mitochondrial function and therefore energy delivery mechanisms. However, I was intrigued to discover that magnesium is also essential to activate immunity against EBV.[84] – 'The authors of this paper describe a new disease, now named X-linked immunodeficiency with magnesium defect, EBV infection, and neoplasia' (XMEN) disease.

Historical note: The Epstein–Barr virus is named after Michael Anthony Epstein (born 18 May 1921), now a professor emeritus at the University of Bristol, and Yvonne Barr (1932–2016), a 1966 PhD graduate from the University of London. Together they discovered the existence of the virus. In 1961, Epstein attended a lecture on 'The Commonest Children's Cancer in Tropical Africa—A Hitherto Unrecognised Syndrome'. This lecture was given by Denis Parsons Burkitt (the cancer he gave this lecture on now bears his name – Burkitt's lymphoma). Burkitt was a surgeon practising in Uganda, and in 1963, a specimen was sent from Uganda to Middlesex Hospital to be cultured. Virus particles were identified in the cultured cells, and the results were published in *The Lancet* in 1964 by Epstein, Bert Achong, and Barr.[85] It is telling that EBV was discovered after investigating a common cancer.

Shingles and chicken pox

I have several patients with post-viral fatigue following these infections. Again, we need to ask if the immune system is activated against such, and again Elispot tests are likely to yield the most useful results as they are both specific and sensitive.

The treatment is the same as for EBV.

Other herpes viruses

If there are ongoing symptoms and positive Elispot tests, or high antibody titres, then I would treat as above.

For oral and genital herpes, topical iodine is a great treatment. Use *ad lib*.

Chapter 33

Lyme disease
(*Borellia burgdorferi*)

If you have skipped straight to this page, then I again iterate: first improve the defences. The starting point, as always, should be Groundhog Acute (page 110), moving on to Groundhog Chronic (page 174). Hit 'em early; hit 'em hard!

There has been a lot of talk in this book about the humble ground hog (*Marmota monax*) but what is she? She is often referred to as a 'woodchuck', but is totally unrelated to wood or chucking – the groundhog does not chuck wood! Instead, this name for the groundhog stems from a Native American (Algonquian (possibly Narragansett)) name for the animal, *'wuchak'*. The similarity between the words has led to the popular tongue-twister:

How much wood would a woodchuck chuck
if a woodchuck could chuck wood?
A woodchuck would chuck all the wood she could chuck
if a woodchuck could chuck wood.

The inclusion of the word 'if' in the second line is now understood but perhaps a more correct, if less entertaining, version of the tongue-twister might be: 'How much wood would a woodchuck chuck … None!' Of course, 'Groundhog' in this book is named for the repetitive loop of the film *Groundhog Day*. We have to repeat these regimes daily to ensure good health.

Why the name *Borellia burgdorferi*?

The bacterial species of the spirochete class of the genus *Borrelia* is so named after two scientists:

- the genus *Borrelia* is named after Amédée Marie Vincent Borrel (1867 – 1936), a French biologist who is credited with pioneering work on the viral theory of cancer. He co-published the treatise *Le microbe de la peste à bubons* concerning the plague bacillus.
- *burgdorferi* is named after the researcher Willy Burgdorfer, who first isolated the bacterium in 1982. Wilhelm 'Willy' Burgdorfer (1925 – 2014) was an American scientist whose work concerned the interactions between animal and human disease agents and their transmitting arthropod (insect etc) vectors.

Diagnosing Lyme disease

Lyme disease, like syphilis (both are caused by spirochetes), is the great mimic. It can produce virtually any pathology. Anybody with almost any neurological disease (dementia, Parkinson's disease, motor neurone disease, multiple sclerosis) could be harbouring *Borrelia*. Consequently, a diagnosis can never be made simply from a list of symptoms and signs, but only from testing. Because this little wretch hides inside body tissues and behind biofilm (see below), this renders many tests unreliable. Do not trust the negative results of antibody tests. The most reliable test is the Elispot test available from Armin labs through https://naturalhealthworldwide.com/ because this has the highest degree of sensitivity and specificity.

Having got a positive result, then recognise that infections rarely come alone.

When sorrows come, they come not single spies, but in battalions.

Claudius in *Hamlet*, Act IV, Scene V,
by William Shakespeare (1564 – 1616)

The longer one has been ill, the more likely it is that there will be another co-infection. This is because if the defences are down in such a way as to allow one infection in, then others will also move in for the same reasons. It is a bit like cancer – the biggest risk for cancer is having one previously. It may well be that you have a cocktail of infections and all need to be treated to get a clinical result. However, my guess is that with Groundhog Chronic (page 110) in place we can tackle these one at a time. This will at least reduce the potential for unpleasant Herxheimer reactions (see page 110). The important point to grasp here is that if Groundhog Chronic is not in place, then you risk becoming re-infected with the very microbe you have just got rid of.

Treatment of Lyme disease

I would always start with the most benign treatments. There is no point fighting with an Exocet missile when a sniper will do – the potential for harm is high. Start with the PK diet, micronutrients, vitamin C, improving energy delivery mechanisms, heat, light… it's Groundhog again (that pesky rodent). Then tackle biofilm and move onto herbals. If one is not seeing clinical progress then, yes, you may have to add in antibiotics.

Biofilm

One defence that microbes employ is to use a protective shield behind which they can hide. The best example of this is dental plaque – a tough crusty deposit that sticks to teeth under which *Streptococcus mutans* makes itself comfortable so that it can attack our teeth and gums. When I was at medical school I was fascinated by a substance called amyloid. This appeared in many different pathologies, from dementias and degenerative conditions to heart disease and cancer, but the reason for its presence was a mystery. We now know many of these conditions are driven by infection – indeed, there is evidence of Lyme involvement in all of these. Put this the other way around – it may be that amyloid is a marker of chronic infection and anyone with this should be fully investigated accordingly for *Borrelia*, *Bartonella*, *Babesia*, *Mycoplasma* and other such. Amyloid (no – it is not 'starch-like' as the name might suggest) is formed of aggregates of prion proteins and these are present in many neurological diseases, such as Alzheimer's, Parkinson's, multiple sclerosis, motor neurone disease and Creutzfeldt-Jakob disease. Indeed, amyloid is found with *Bartonella*, *Babesia*, *Chlamydia*, *Yersinia*, *Ehrlichia*, Epstein Barr virus, herpes I, herpes zoster, roseola, HIV, hepatitis C, cytomegalovirus… and many other such.

Remember: we know that the brain clears amyloid during non-REM sleep. It may be that this is part of a more general clear-out of infectious microbes. Non-REM sleep is essential for life. Make sure you get it. See Chapter 6 for the references on non-REM sleep (page 222).

Dr David Horowitz, a Lyme disease expert, maintains that this biofilm needs to be attacked with the enzyme serrapeptidase. We know this enzyme can render MRSA more susceptible to antibiotics, so it is a least biologically plausible that it may help. Serrapeptidase may additionally help reduce microbes in the upper gut and perhaps break down fibrin clots behind which infections lurk. I am not sure how important this intervention is, but one can do no harm with it. The dose is serrapeptidase 160,000 iu (international units) three times daily.

Kill the microbes with herbals

I have taken the following recommendations from the work of the medical herbalist Steven Buhner and other doctors, such as Andrew Wright. Dr Wright is another one of those doctors who has been hounded by the General Medical Council for trusting his patients and trying to treat their Lyme disease. Firstly, we need to use herbs as per Chapter 13 to improve the defences – namely, *Astragalus*, rhodiola and *Cordyceps*.

Secondly, we should use herbs to kill *Borrelia* directly. The doses given below are the high doses recommended by Chinese medicine. You may not need the full dose. Adjust according to your response. You may initially experience Herxheimer, or 'die off' reactions, with worsening of symptoms (see page 234). The idea is that 'Herxing' is some sort of allergic reaction to the dead microbes. This is biologically plausible. If microbes are hidden away behind biofilm, then as they break up, fragments spill out and the immune system attacks them. If such a reaction is severe, reduce the dose, allow improvement and then try to crank the dose up again. This is where you need to manage your own treatment day by day and listen to your symptoms. Once you have recovered and symptoms have resolved, continue with treatment for at least two months. Most people need eight to 12 months of treatment to recover. Some need low dose treatment long term, perhaps for life.

Table 33.1: Herbs that will fight *Borrelia*

Herb	Form and maximum dose	Notes
Japanese knotweed, also known as resveratrol, which is the active ingredient (not the grape stuff – must be knotweed)	Root powder – gradually build up to one tablespoon taken three times daily OR knotweed resveratrol capsules 500 mg – build up to 16 daily	Like any effective treatment, a Herxheimer reaction may occur. Thins the blood, so stop using if you need surgery and take care if taking blood thinners
Cats claw	Root powder 1500 mg taken four times daily OR Capsules 500 mg x 12 daily Some people just need one capsule taken three times daily	Very safe May thin the blood so stop using if you need surgery and take care if taking blood thinners
Andrographis	Very bitter, so use the capsules Up to 600 mg x 2, three times daily	Start with a low dose as it may cause hives. (My guess is that putting in place all the Groundhog interventions may prevent this)

One of the joys of using herbs is that they attack microbes in a multiplicity of ways. This makes it much harder for resistant strains of Lyme to evolve and reduces the chances of antibiotic resistance developing.

Kill the microbes with antibiotics

I do not pretend any great experience of treating Lyme and the following recommendations come from Dr Richard Horowitz's book, *How Can I Get Better?*[86]

Having got all the above in place, if you are not seeing a clinical result, you have to consider antimicrobials to kill Lyme and other co-infections. In dealing with them we have to take a 'tuberculosis-like' approach – that is, it is combinations of antibiotics that will get the result, and these have to be taken over months, not weeks. Combinations of antibiotics further illustrate the arms race approach – the more different ways one can attack, the better. Furthermore, combinations make it more difficult for resistant strains of bacteria to appear because they would have to simultaneously evolve two or three different mechanisms for drug resistance.

Dr Horowitz often uses intravenous antibiotics. I have not included those regimens simply because they are almost always impossible to put in place in the UK. However, I hope, and believe, that putting in the above to improve the defences will make the oral regimes as effective as the intravenous ones. It is important to combine antimicrobials for 'cell wall' and 'cystic' forms of Lyme together with those to get at intracellular microbes. With Lyme and co-infections, the microbes do not exist in one form – they exist in a 'cell wall' form but once established in the body they cycle between 'cell wall' forms and 'cystic' forms.

The oral regimes of antibiotics he recommends are as follows. For:
- Cell wall forms: co-amoxiclav 500/125, two capsules taken three times daily
- Cystic forms: metronidazole 400 mg, three times daily
- Intracellular location: doxycycline 100 mg, twice daily

Other oral antibiotics that can be used for the same durations as above if there is intolerance to medications or poor clinical response to treatment are as follows. For:
- Cell wall forms: cefuroxime 500 mg, twice daily
- Cystic forms: tinidazole 400 mg, three times daily
- Intracellular location: azithromycin 500 mg, once daily, or ciproxin 500 mg, twice daily (Be mindful that ciproxin can cause tendon damage – any pain and stop it at once).

Duration of treatment

Horowitz recommends that treatment should be given for at least two months, and continued for two months after the patient is symptom free. This may be possible at a lower rate of dosing. My limited experience is that eight to 12 months of treatment is required.

Some practitioners advocate 'pulsing' (intermittent use) of antimicrobials. I cannot see the logic of this. If we are fighting a war, then we want all our resources employed all at once – scorched earth policy, foot soldiers, cavalry, machine guns, bombs, the lot. I am quite sure Wellington would not have chosen to give Napoleon a bit of a break during the battle of Waterloo!

At the same time, protect the microbiome from antibiotic damage – see Chapter 37.

Response to treatment

This can be monitored clinically ('how do you feel?') and also with Elispot blood tests to show (we hope!) that the white cells are reacting less against the microbes as the numbers (of microbes) come down. However, in the short term Elispot results may be more positive as the microbes are killed and the dead parts come out of hiding.

As always, the clinical response should be your best guide, or to put it another way:

The proof of the pudding is in the eating.

14th Century English Proverb – possibly earlier, where it was known as:

Jt is ywrite that euery thing Hymself sheweth in the tastyng
The shorter form 'the proof is in the pudding', which dates back to the 1920s and came into common use in the United States in the 1950s, is becoming increasingly popular, although keeping a proof in a pudding might be messy!

If you are not seeing the expected improvements, then consider the possibility that there may be other infections… read on!

Chapter 34

Bartonella and *Babesia*

Bartonella species have been infecting humans for thousands of years, evidenced by *Bartonella quintana* DNA found in a 4000-year-old tooth.[87] The genus is named after Alberto Leonardo Barton Thompson (1871–1950), a Peruvian microbiologist who discovered the aetiologic agent of Carrion´s disease. The bacterium was named *Bartonella bacilliformis*. It is the type species of the genus *Bartonella*, and family Bartonellaceae.

Bartonella is much more common than we think – it is transmitted by biting insects and animals through contaminated bites or scratches (hence 'cat scratch fever'). Many pets carry *Bartonella*. In Germany a study of 270 healthy adults found 30% to be infected with *Bartonella*; in Greece a study of 50 healthy people found 20% to be infected, (I have to say I wonder how the researchers defined 'healthy'!); and in Spain a study of 83 cat owners showed 30% to be infected.

The point of this is that it is clear that this 'infection' is very common but most people do not know they have it. The difference between being an asymptomatic carrier and a sufferer is one's own defences. Modern Western lifestyles are gorgeous – I would not wish to live at any other time or place in history. But again, we are unwittingly eroding our immune system through these very Western diets and lifestyles (but we can make choices!).

Furthermore, climate change means blood-sucking insects can move into new, warm habitats and take advantage of a new group of naïve, relatively defenceless mammal hosts – see the paper by Sabine Nooten, Nigel R. Andrew, and Lesley Hughes.[88] Interestingly this study showed that the structure of the herbivorous insect community was less affected by climate change effects than was the non-herbivorous insect community, thus strengthening the view that mammal hosts are at significant risk.

Bartonella is one of the early microbes to take full advantage of this tourist honey pot. We cannot possibly eradicate it with antimicrobials, but we can make our own bodies such an uncomfortable and difficult place to live that it cannot flourish there.

We also know that *Bartonella* can cause severe disease if our natural defences are compromised – the classic clinical pictures can be seen in patients immunosuppressed by drugs or HIV, and are typically chronic fatigue with additional symptoms of systemic inflammation (fever, lymphadenopathy, neurological and psychiatric symptoms, muscle and joint symptoms etc). It colonises four sites: red blood cells, spleen, liver, and bone marrow, and from there moves into the lining of blood vessels. Thus, like *Borrelia*, it could produce almost any symptom, including organ damage or organ failure.

Diagnosis

Again, as with Lyme, one can never make the diagnosis simply from a list of symptoms and signs; one can only make the diagnosis from testing. Many tests are unreliable. Do not trust the negative results of antibody tests. The most reliable test, as with *Borrelia*, is the Elispot test available from Armin labs through https://naturalhealthworldwide.com because this has the highest degree of sensitivity and specificity.

Treatment

A patient with established *Bartonella* will need serious bombs in order to reduce the numbers of *Bartonella* so that their own immune system can take over to control things in the longer term. Depending on the severity of the clinical and laboratory results one may choose to start with herbals or prescription drugs.

Herbal treatments

These largely work through improving defences and indirect killing rather than direct killing of *Bartonella*.

Table 34.1: Herbs for treating *Bartonella*

Herb	Form and maximum dose	Notes
Groundhog herbs of *Astragalus*, rhodiola and *Cordyceps*	See Chapter 13	
Japanese knotweed, also known as resveratrol (not the grape stuff – must be knotweed)	Root powder – gradually build up to one tablespoon taken three times daily OR Knotweed resveratrol capsules 500 mg – build up to 16 daily	*Bartonella* kill does not apparently result in Herxheimer reactions. (This suggests to me that biofilm is not an issue)
Chinese skullcap	Root powder – build up to 3 grams taken three times daily	Additionally effective against herpes viruses, *Mycoplasma*, *Rickettsia*, *Yersinia*. This herb seems like a jolly good all-rounder!

Antibiotic treatments

Again, the best results come from combinations of antibiotics given over months – typically eight months to two years for sufficient bacterial clearance. However, my guess is that if combined with Groundhog Chronic and the above herbals (also as part of Groundhog Chronic), the dose and duration could be substantially reduced. A typical antibiotic regime would start with doxycycline 100 mg twice daily with azithromycin 500 mg once daily. Again, I would wish to continue treatment for two months after symptoms had settled.

Remember treatment will never clear every last microbe – some sneaky wretches will be hidden away, so back to Groundhog Chronic to prevent recurrence.

Babesia

The *Babesia* organism is named after Viktor Babès, who first recognised it in the blood cells of cattle in the late 19th century. Babesiosis is the name of the disease caused by infection with *Babesia*.

Babès (1854 – 1926) was a Romanian physician, bacteriologist, academician and professor who co-authored one of the first treatises of bacteriology in the world – 'Bacteria and their role in pathological anatomy and histology of infectious diseases'. In early life, Babès was most interested in poetry, music and literature, and excelled at sport and dramatics. In fact he began his academic career by studying the dramatic arts in Budapest. But the death of his sister, Alma, caused by tuberculosis, at a young age, led him to abandon his dramatic arts studies and enrol to study medicine.

Babesia is a malaria-like parasite. It too lives in red blood cells. It has been found in virtually all species of animals, although classically it is passed on by ticks. It is very likely that other biting insects can also transmit it. It can be passed on in blood products and there is one reported case of transplacental spread. Many 'healthy' people harbour *Babesia*. It is an ancient organism that humans have been living with for millions of years and we are dependent on our immune system to keep it under control.

In fact, possibly the first reference to babesiosis is in the book of *Exodus*, which alludes to a plague of 'murrain', which affected cattle, camels, sheep and other domestic animals but more recently we have the excellent paper 'Babesiosis: Recent insights into an ancient disease' by KP Hunfeld et al.[89]

An acute infection will result in a 'flu-like illness (mini-malaria) and possibly haemolytic (involving the rupture or destruction of red blood cells) anaemia. As with Lyme, this may be followed with an outbreak of arthritis and possibly chronic symptoms of fatigue – that is to say, chronic fatigue syndrome or ME.

Diagnosis

Babesia parasites may be seen in a blood under a microscope as a pathogical 'Maltese Cross' in red blood cells. One cannot rely on clinical pictures to make or refute the diagnosis – you have to have a high index of suspicion and do the tests. Again, antibody testing is unreliable. Elispot testing has the best sensitivity and specificity. Because the infection affects the blood, there may be other clues from routine blood testing, such as low red cell count, low white cell count, low platelets and liver or kidney damage.

Treatment

Table 34.2: Herbs and prescription drugs for treating *Babesia*

Herb	Form and maximum dose	Notes
Groundhog herbs of *Astragalus*, rhodiola and *Cordyceps*	See Chapter 13	
Artemisinin	As capsules 200 mg taken three times daily	Of proven benefit in the treatment of malaria
Atovaquone AND	750 mg twice daily for at least 10 days, possibly longer depending on the symptoms	
Azithromycin	500 mg twice daily for at least 10 days, possibly longer depending on the clinical response	

Philosophical note by Craig: Like Crohn (Chapter 31), Babès was motivated into a medical career by family medical concerns. Both these men possessed considerable talents in many spheres of human endeavour. It can seem very random how events determine the paths we choose, and I do worry that modern life closes the opportunities for such Renaissance men and women. Sarah gave me a book *The Last Man Who Knew Everything*, a biography of Thomas Young. It has the sub-title *Thomas Young, the Anonymous Polymath Who Proved Newton Wrong, Explained How We See, Cured the Sick and Deciphered the Rosetta Stone*. Maybe there is more to know nowadays, and I am being a pessimist, or maybe the way we learn and 'teach' our children reduces the chances of the polymath being able to rise to the surface these days, but whichever, I think that such people are rarer than they used to be. This is a shame, culturally, and is also detrimental to the advancement of human knowledge. It is the crossover of intellectual disciplines that yields the eureka moments, and becoming ever more specialised in ever narrower fields reduces the possibilities of those inspirational moments.

Education is the kindling of a flame, not the filling of a vessel.
Socrates (470 – 399 BC (approx))

Chapter 35

Mycoplasma and *Chlamydia*

Mycoplasma

The name '*Mycoplasma*' derives from the Greek μυκής, 'mykes' (fungus), and πλάσμα, 'plasma' (formed). This term was first used by Albert Bernhard Frank (a German botanist, 1839 – 1900) in 1889 to describe a state of plant cell cytoplasm in which there had been infiltration from fungus-like micro-organisms. Later Julian Nowak ((1865 – 1946), a Polish microbiologist and politician who served as prime minister of Poland in 1922, put forward the genus name *Mycoplasma* for micro-organisms which were visible with a microscope but which passed through filters impermeable to bacteria. *Mycoplasma* species are, indeed, the smallest free-living organisms. (Viruses cannot live independently of a host cell.)

The same issues that apply to *Bartonella* and are described in Chapter 34, also apply to *Mycoplasma* and we are seeing epidemics of such because we are losing the arms race. Those individuals who have the intelligence to see this and, more importantly, the determination to put in place the defences before Armageddon strikes, will survive in the longer term. Even with our more virulent plagues, such as the Black Death which killed one third of the population of Europe in the mid 14th century, two thirds survived. For whatever reason, those survivors had the necessary defences in place. I know for sure that the modern-day plagues have arrived and I do not want to leave my defences to Lady Luck.

The personification of luck as female has its roots in Fortuna, the Roman goddess of fortune; this was a capricious form of luck, though. Fortuna might bring good

> or bad luck; she was often represented as blind or veiled to the woes of man. This imagery carries forward to modern depictions of Lady Justice, who is blindfolded because of her impartiality in the administration of the law.

Mycoplasmas are so damned versatile and clever that they can inhabit not just mammals and reptiles, but also fish, insects and plants. Whilst we may be aware of the sexually transmitted *Mycoplasma*, the organism can be spread by biting insects and by ingestion and inhalation. *Mycoplasmas* are a well-recognised cause of pelvic inflammatory disease, miscarriage and atypical pneumonia, but they can infect any organ and drive diseases such as rheumatoid arthritis, Hodgkin's disease, neurological disease (Tourette's, Guillain-Barre, motor neurone disease, psychosis, seizures and other such). Please see the reference section (page 229) for references to relevant medical papers.[90, 91, 92, 93, 94, 95]

I heard about *Mycoplasma fermentans* because of my interest in Gulf War syndrome (GWS). GWS has been closely linked to vaccination and exposure to organophosphates. Fifty per cent of Gulf War veterans tested positive for *M. fermentans* (almost certainly used in biological warfare). It is biologically plausible to see how these A1 fit troops had their immune system compromised, which allowed *Mycoplasma* to invade. Gulf War veterans subsequently suffered high rates of neurological disease, especially Parkinson's and motor neurone disease (MND, also known as ALS – amyotrophic lateral sclerosis). I know this because I have seen and treated them. Indeed, one study showed that 90% of MND sufferers tested positive for *Mycoplasma*. Like other *Mycoplasmas*, *M. fermentans* is characterised by lack of a peptidoglycan cell wall and this results in resistance to many but not all antibacterial agents.

When these Gulf War veterans returned home, their previously healthy families developed diseases. In particular, their children developed autism. Indeed, 58% of autistic children will test positive for *Mycoplasma* (29% test positive for HHV6 and 8.3% for *Chlamydia pneumoniae*). The vaccination link to autism could be explained by a simple infection hypothesis since *M. fermentans* now contaminates all cell cultures, including those used for vaccines. So, vaccinating children may give them a dose of *M. fermentans* and it is possibly this infectious agent that causes autism.

Mycoplasma is a common co-infection – if you have tested positive for Lyme you have a 70% chance of being additionally infected with *Mycoplasma*.

Diagnosis

Mycoplasma can be picked up via my four Gs – 'gobs and guts, genitals and gnats'. If you were a betting person and your ME sufferer was not recovering with Groundhog Chronic, you would put your money on *Mycoplasma* as the misery agent. Because it is so ubiquitous and so pernicious, you simply must have a high index of diagnostic suspicion. For example, *Mycoplasma* should be included in the differential diagnosis of:

- Airways: pneumonia, bronchitis, pharyngitis, rhinitis, earaches, sinusitis
- Gut: hepatitis, pancreatitis
- Joints: arthritis, arthralgias, myalgias, polyarthritis
- Kidneys: glomerulonephritis
- Eye: uveitis
- Brain: myelitis, Guillain-Barré syndrome, encephalitis, meningitis, polyradiculopathy, peripheral facial paresis, optical neuritis, haemorrhagic leukoencephalitis, peripheral polyneuropathy, cranial nerve neuritis, radiculitis
- Autoimmunity.

Again, IgG and IgM antibodies can be misleading, but Elispot has a high level of sensitivity and specificity. As described earlier, these tests are available at Armin laboratories through https://naturalhealthworldwide.com/

Chlamydia

I have lumped *Chlamydia* together with *Mycoplasma* because the treatment is the same. *Chlamydia* appears clinically as follows:

- 'Gobs and guts': it may present with respiratory symptoms, including pneumonia (*Chlamydia pneumoniae*)
- 'Genitals': it is a sexually transmitted disease (*Chlamydia trachomatis*), which may spread to cause eye inflammation, initially conjunctivitis but then the blinding disease trachoma
- 'Gnats': it is theoretically possible to be transmitted by insect bites.

Diagnosis

Both *C. trachomatis* and *C. pneumoniae* can be diagnosed by Elispot testing at Armin labs.

Treatment of *Mycoplasma* and *Chlamydia*

Groundhog Chronic (page 174 plus Chapters 27, 28 and 29) and:

Herbal treatments

Table 35.1: Herbs to kill *Mycoplasma* and *Chlamydia*

Herb	Form and maximum dose	Notes
Cordyceps, rhodiola and *Astragalus*, as per 'improving the defences' (see Chapter 13)	See Chapter 13	See Chapter 13
Chinese skullcap	Root powder – build up to 3 grams taken three times daily (total of 9 grams)	Additionally effective against herpes viruses, *Rickettsia* and *Yersinia*

Antibiotic treatments

The regimes are the same as for *Bartonella* so what I say below is a repeat prescription. Skip this if you have already consumed it… again, the best results come from combinations of antibiotics given over months – typically, eight months to two years for complete bacterial clearance. However, my guess is that if combined with Groundhog and the above herbals, the dose and duration could be substantially reduced.

A typical antibiotic regime would start with:
- doxycycline 100 mg twice daily, with
- azithromycin 500 mg, once daily.

Again, I would wish to continue treatment for two months after symptoms have settled.

Once cleared, carry on with Groundhog Chronic to prevent recurrence.

Chapter 36

Rickettsia (*Ehrlichia* and *Anaplasma*) and *Yersinia*

Rickettsia microbes are known to cause seriously nasty acute infections, such as typhus fever (not typhoid). During the Napoleonic wars and the French retreat from Moscow, more French soldiers died of typhus than were killed by the Russians. Anne Frank died aged 15 at Bergen-Belsen concentration camp from typhus. Epidemics continue to date. It is spread by lice and fleas, including those of our pet dogs and cats.

Yersinia in its acute form again causes serous disease. The Black Death (*Yersinia pestis*) between 1347 and 1352 killed at least one third of the European population. In the late 19th century it arrived in China where it killed ten million people. It is spread by rats and their fleas. It was called the 'Black' Death because of the dark patches on the skin caused by subcutaneous bleeding.

Some say that the nursery rhyme (or folksong, or playground singing game) 'Ring a Ring o' Roses' (or 'Ring Around the Rosie', or 'Ring a Ring o' Rosie') is about the Black Death (where the 'pocketful of posies' could be something to ward off the disease or even to cover the stench of sickness, or maybe to be placed on the graves of loved ones) but folklorists reject this idea – you can find a discussion at www.snopes.com/language/literary/rosie.asp

These microbes are clever little sods. They hijack fleas and other biting insects, so bites bypass normal skin barriers. *Yersinia* interferes with normal immune responses to invaders by inhibiting phagocytosis (white cells gobbling up foreign cells), interfering with immune signalling and hiding inside white cells (monocytes). *Rickettsia* possesses lengths of DNA identical to mitochondrial DNA. Indeed, it may be that mitochondria and *Rickettsia* have similar ancestry. *Rickettsia* primarily infects the lining of blood vessels and, like *Yersinia*, inhibits host defences.

As with so many 'stealth' infections, there is an acute phase with a 'flu-like illness which, if one survives, may progress on to a chronic phase. Again, these chronic phases do not have a characteristic clinical picture of symptoms and signs. The clinical picture may be ME/fibromyalgia, or it may involve organ failure (dementia, heart disease, kidney or liver disease etc). Symptoms and signs are so often wrongly attributed to other causes, such as age, arteriosclerosis or 'degeneration' without proper thought going into the causes of such.

Diagnosis

To have any chance of diagnosing these conditions one needs a high index of suspicion. Do not rely on a history of tick bites or flea bites. Do not rely on the person not being in an endemic area. Do not rely on classical pathological lesions. Mildly abnormal haematology or liver function tests may be a clue. Be a nasty, suspicious, inquiring, 'never say die' person and be prepared to splash out some cash on proper testing. It may be the best investment you ever make in your health! (See Chapter 28, page 163.) Again, IgG and IgM antibodies can be misleading but Elispot has a high level of sensitivity and specificity. As before, these tests are available at Armin laboratories through https://naturalhealthworldwide.com/

Treatment of *Rickettsia* (*Ehrlichia* and *Anaplasma*) and *Yersinia*

Combine the following with Groundhog Chronic (page 174, plus Chapters 27, 28 and 29).

Table 36.1: Herbs and prescription drugs to kill *Rickettsia* and *Yersinia*

Herbs/drugs	Form and maximum dose	Notes
Cordyceps, rhodiola and *Astragalus* – as per 'improving the defences' (see Chapter 13)	See Chapter 13	See Chapter 13
Chinese skullcap	Root powder – build up to 3 grams taken three times daily (total of 9 grams)	Additionally effective against herpes viruses and *Mycoplasma*
Doxycycline AND	100 mg twice daily	I would recommend combinations of antibiotics given over months – typically eight months to two years. I would wish to continue treatment for two months after symptoms have settled
Azithromycin	500 mg daily	Ditto above

Once cleared, carry on with Groundhog Chronic to prevent recurrence.

Chapter 37

Preventing antibiotic damage to the gut microbiome

Preventing antibiotic damage to the gut microbiome is a question that many flag up, and with good reason. We know that antibiotics are potentially highly damaging to the gut microbiome and I see many patients whose illness has clearly been made worse or even triggered by antibiotics. On the flip side I see many patients who only feel well taking antibiotics. I would not like to practise medicine without using these drugs!

How do we get the best of both worlds? No-one really knows the answer to this question, but the good news is that the microbiome is very stable. Potential problems with antibiotics occur in the lower gut, or colon, where the microbiome resides. If you eat a PK diet (high fat, high fibre – see page 236), this is highly protective against antibiotic damage for the following reasons:

1. Antibiotics are fairly well absorbed in the upper gut. This department should be near sterile and so the potential for harm here is minimal. Where there is no upper fermenting gut (remember microbes can only ferment sugar and carbs), absorption of antibiotic will be more efficient. This means there is less to pass downstream into the colon.

2. Some antibiotic will get into the colon but its concentration is diluted by the large numbers of microbes, high volume of fibre and the water that this draws into the gut. With antibiotic kill it is a numbers game.

3. A high-fibre diet results in a bulky stool with short gut transit time so antibiotics do not spend so much time in the gut. By contrast, it is more likely that the constipated patient will see adverse effects from antibiotics.

4. A high-fibre PK diet feeds microbes. Given the right food, microbes can double

their numbers every 20 minutes. Even if numbers are knocked back by antibiotics, they will recover quickly.

What this means is that, contrary to popular opinion, taking some probiotic capsules alone may not suffice. To protect the microbiome during antibiotic therapy we need to tip the scales in our favour:

1. Eat a PK diet, rich in prebiotics and high in vegetable fibre and dirty vegetables – lots of them!
2. Eat live, actively fermenting, probiotic cultures such as kefir and sauerkraut – lots of it!
3. Take vitamin C to bowel tolerance. We know this kills friendly bacteria as well as unfriendly, but again it is a numbers game. With the PK diet, the friendlies are far more abundant than the unfriendlies. There is an important synergism between vitamin C and antibiotics whereby vitamin C enhances the effect of antibiotics and protects against side effects; this is illustrated by the previously mentioned Marik study which reduced mortality from septicaemia from 40% to 1% when vitamin C was added in to the antibiotic regime.[96]

Some doctors routinely advocate antifungal drugs when antibiotics are used. My rules of the game are as follows:

- If the patient is particularly prone to thrush, then I would prescribe an antifungal such as itraconazole 100 mg daily or fluconazole 50 mg daily for the duration of the antibiotic course plus another two days. (These can be purchased over the counter at a chemist in the UK.) For many, herbal preparations such as high-dose garlic (allicin), caprylic acid (coconut oil) or plant tannins work well.
- If the patient is not prone to fungal infections, then I would not prescribe an antifungal. My experience is that if Groundhog is in place (see Chapter 15, page 98), fungal infections or fermentations are preventable. Yeast can only ferment sugar and digested starches. The low-carb diet means they cannot grow.

Antifungal medications

Approximately 1% of the normal microbiome is comprised of yeasts and these should be present in the colon. Consequently, the potential for antifungals to cause damage to the microbiome is minimal for all the reasons given above. This is supported by a wealth of clinical experience. Doctors like me have been using antifungals to treat 'candida' problems for decades with no serious complications.

Antiviral medication

Generally 15% of the microbiome is viral. These viruses do not attack human cells because their host is bacterial – they eat bacteria and so are called 'bacteriophages'. The microbiome too is an ecosystem with its own predator-prey relationships.

Big fleas have little fleas, on their back to bite 'em
Little fleas have lesser fleas and so ad infinitum.

The Siphonaptera (nursery rhyme)

Some credit the basis for this nursery rhyme to Jonathan Swift (author of *Gulliver's Travels*, 1667 – 1745), from his long satirical poem *On Poetry: a Rhapsody* (1733). Here is the relevant excerpt:

The vermin only teaze and pinch
Their foes superior by an inch.
So, naturalists observe, a flea
Has smaller fleas that on him prey;
And these have smaller still to bite 'em,
And so proceed ad infinitum.

Do antiviral drugs upset bacteriophages? I do not know, but I doubt it. I say that partly from clinical experience and partly from biological plausibility – antivirals have specific actions and are specific to groups of viruses. My guess is that bacteriophages are sufficiently different from viruses that infect humans for this not to be problem.

Chapter 38

Other infections

This book cannot possibly address all the known infectious causes of disease. There are many I have not included, either because they are rare or because we do not have specific antimicrobials. We can treat these only with Groundhog Chronic. However, that is of proven benefit. Good immune defences explain why not everyone died from the Black Death or Spanish 'flu, not everyone became paralysed after contracting polio and not everyone develops a post-viral chronic fatigue syndrome after glandular fever.

I do hope my ME patients will forgive me for not including a detailed analysis of ME triggered by polio (either the disease or the vaccine), coxsackie A and B viruses, ECHO virus, enterovirus 71, Bornholm and influenza viruses. The fact of the matter is that many of my patients whose illness has clearly been triggered by such recover very well with all the 'improving the defences' interventions of Groundhog Chronic (page 174). The body wants to be well; give it half a chance and it will recover.

Just do it.

Part V

Be prepared for the kill

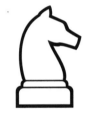

Appendix 1

The battle first-aid box

John Churchill, 1st Duke of Blenheim (26 May 1650 – 16 June 1722) was a successful general, partly because he made sure his armies were fully equipped for battle. The essence of success is to be prepared with the necessary to combat all unwanted boarders. Strike early and strike hard.

Of John Churchill, Captain Robert Parker (who was at the Battle of Blenheim, 13 August 1704) wrote: '… it cannot be said that he ever slipped an opportunity of fighting…' We must be equally belligerent in our own individual battles, and part of this belligerence is preparedness, so keep the following in your own 'battle first-aid box' and use it at the first sign of attack.

Table A2.1: What to keep at the ready in your battle first-aid box

For acute infections	Vitamin C as ascorbic acid – at least 500 grams (It is its own preservative so lasts for years) Lugol's iodine 12% – at least 50 ml (It is its own preservative so lasts for years) Iodoral tablets 12.5 mg Bee Prepared (page 218) Zinc and vitamin C lozenges Echinacea
Conjunctivitis – indeed, any eye infection	Iodine eye drops e.g. Minims povidine iodine 5% OR Lugol's iodine 12% (2 drops in 5 ml of water); this does not sting the eyes and is the best killer of all microbes in the eye
Upper airways infections	Lugol's iodine to use in steam inhalation OR in a salt pipe (drizzle in 4 drops of Lugol's iodine 12% per dose)
Skin breaches	Salt – 2 teaspoonfuls (10 grams) in 500 ml water (approx 1 pint), plus Lugol's iodine 12% (20 ml) – use *ad lib* to wash any wound; once clean, allow to dry Iodine ointment 10% to smother the wound Plaster or micropore to protect
Fractures	If the skin is broken, treat the wound as above Immobilise If a limb fracture, wrap in cotton wool to protect the limb, bandage abundantly with vet wrap to splint it Then the next stop is … casualty
Burns	As for breaches of the skin If a large burn, then use cling film to protect it once cleaned (Put iodine ointment on the cling film first, then apply to the burn) Protect as per fractures above, then the next step is A&E
Wounds – sterile dressings	Melolin is a good all-rounder Large roll of cotton wool, crepe bandages (various sizes) and micropore tape to protect any damaged area from further trauma Vet Wrap bandage – this is wonderful stuff, especially if you are in the wilds, to hold everything together (see page 220).

Gastroenteritis	Sunshine salt – to make up a perfect rehydration drink add 5 grams (1 teaspoonful) to 1 litre of water, which gives a 0.5% solution
Urine infections	Multistix to test urine D mannose and potassium citrate
Consider acquiring antibiotics for intelligent use	These should not be necessary if you stick to Groundhog Basic (page 98) and apply Groundhog Acute (page 110) BUT I too live in the real world and am no paragon of virtue, so if you slip off the band wagon:
	Clove oil[97] Amoxil 500 mg x 21 capsules for dental infection
	Cephalexin 500 mg three times daily for ENT and respiratory infections
	Doxycycline 100 mg twice daily for diverticulitis
	Trimethoprim 200 grams twice daily for urinary infection
	If you are susceptible to a particular infection, make sure you always hold the relevant antibiotic. The sooner you start treatment, the less the damage. Always start with Groundhog Acute.

Putting together such a battle first-aid box is as much an intellectual exercise as a practical one and this book, along with our book *Prevent and Cure Diabetes – delicious diets, not dangerous drugs* give such intellectual imperative. As Shakespeare writes in *Henry V*:

All things are ready, if our minds be so.

William Shakespeare (1564 – 23 April 1616)

Appendix 2

Recommended products

Daylong pressure garments
To prevent deep vein thrombosis
www.daylong.co.uk/shop-by-brand/medi.html?gclid=EAIaIQobChMInq-hkvXe1wIVyrft
Ch05gQD3EAAYASAAEgKuL_D_BwE

D-mannose
One typical product is:
https://uk.iherb.com/pr/Now-Foods-D-Mannose-500-mg-120-Veggie-Caps/525 – take 3
x 500 mg capsules one to three times a day

Electro-smog
For products to diagnose and treat:
www.healthy-house.co.uk/electro
http://drmyhill.co.uk/wiki/Electrical_sensitivity

Herbs
UK – www.indigo-herbs.co.uk
UK – www.hybridherbs.co.uk
USA – www.mountainroseherbs.com

Immune support
Bee Prepared – contains bee propolis, astaxanthin, olive leaf, Reishi mushrooms and
elderberry – www.unbeelievablehealth.co.uk

Iodine products

Iodoral can be obtained from
www.amazon.co.uk/Iodoral-12-5-mg-180-tablets/dp/B000X843VG
and other online shops
IodoRx – an equivalent product
www.salesatdrmyhill.co.uk/iodorx-90-tablets-145-p.asp
Lugol's iodine 12%
www.amazon.co.uk/Lugols-Iodine-12-Solution-30ml/dp/B00A25GCLO

Potassium citrate

These are all example products with their respective doses:
- Effervescent tablets (brand Effercitrate) – take two tablets, up to three times a day. Take the tablets dissolved into a whole glassful of water.
- Liquid medicine (brand Cymaclear) – take two 5 ml spoonfuls, stirred into a whole glassful of water. You can take up to three doses a day.
- Sachets (brand Cystopurin) – empty the contents of one sachet into a whole glassful of water. Stir it well before drinking. Take one sachet, three times daily.

Sunshine salt

One teaspoon (5 ml) contains all the minerals and vitamin D needed for one day.
sales@drmyhill.co.uk

Tests and their interpretation

- www.bloodtestsdirect.co.uk/ – where blood tests can be accessed directly without a doctor's request. Many can be done on fingerdrop samples of blood.
- www.arminlabs.com/en – blood tests can be accessed directly without the need for a referral from a doctor or health practitioner.
- www.biolab.co.uk/ – needs referral from a health practitioner – see NHW below.
- www.gdx.net/uk/ – Genova labs for stool, urine and saliva testing – needs referral from a health practitioner – see NHW below.
- Natural Health Worldwide: www.naturalhealthworldwide.com

Urine infection check
Search for 'Multistix' dip sticks
sales@doctormyhill.co.uk

Vet Wrap bandage
Available from many suppliers, eg. www.storkz.com and amazon.co.uk
Be aware Vet Wrap bandage tape contains latex.

Vitamin C
For those with a corn allergy intolerance search for 'ascorbic acid corn free sago palm'
www.pureformulas.com/sagoc500-90-tablets-by-nutri-west.html

Vitamins and non-herbals supplements
UK – www.salesatdrmyhill.co.uk
UK – www.biocare.co.uk
UK – www.naturesbest.co.uk
USA – www.swansonvitamins.com
USA – www.puritan.com

References

Chapter 1: Life is an arms race

1. Taubenberger JK, Morens DM. Influenza: The Once and Future Pandemi. *Public Health Reports* 2010; 125(Suppl 3): 16–26. www.ncbi.nlm.nih.gov/pmc/articles/PMC2862331/

Chapter 2: Infections that drive Western diseases

2. Office for National Statistics. *Deaths Registered in England and Wales 2015.* November 2016. www.ons.gov.uk/peoplepopulationandcommunity/birthsdeathsandmarriages/deaths/bulletins/deathsregisteredinenglandandwalesseriesdr/ 2015
3. Bredesen DE. *Reversal of Cognitive Decline: A novel therapeutic program.* www.doctormyhill.co.uk/drmyhill/images/0/07/Reversal-of-Cognitive-decline-Bredesen.pdf
4. de Flora S, Bonanni P. The prevention of infection-associated cancers. *Carcinogenesis* 2011; 32(6): 787–795. www.ncbi.nlm.nih.gov/pmc/articles/PMC3314281/
5. Berg RD. Bacterial translocation from the gastrointestinal tract. *Adv Exp Med Biol* 1999; 473: 11-30. www.ncbi.nlm.nih.gov/pubmed/1065934
6. Nishihara. Disclosure of the major causes of mental illness—mitochondrial deterioration in brain neurons via opportunistic infection. www.drmyhill.co.uk/drmyhill/images/d/dc/NISHIHARA.pdf

Chapter 4: Your enemy is fiendishly clever

7.   Braun L, Cohen M. *Herbs and Natural Supplements* (2 volumes). 4th edition. Edinburgh: Churchill Livingstone; 2015.

8.   Buhner SH. *Herbal Antibiotics (Medicinal Herb Guide)*. Storey Communications; 2000.

9.   Buhner SH. *Herbal Antivirals.* Storey Publishing; 2013.

10. How M-J, Huang S-H, Chang C-Y, Lin Y-K et al. Baicalein ethylacetate and chloroform extracts of *Scutellaria baicalensis* inhibit the neuraminidase activity of pandemic 2009 H1N1 and seasonal influenza A viruses. *Evidence Based Complementary and Alternative Medicine* 2013; 2013:750803.

11. https://examine.com/supplements/scutellaria-baicalensis

12. Mould J, et al. Influenza B virus BM2 protein has ion channel activity that conducts protons across membranes. *Developmental Cell* 2003; 5(1):175-184. DOI: 1016/S1534-5807(03)00190-4.

13. Atkinson SK, Sadofsky LR, Morice AH. How does rhinovirus cause the common cold cough? *BMJ Open Respiratory Research* 2016; 3(1):e000118.

14. A good starting point for information about the 'Spanish' 'flu epidemic is: https://en.wikipedia.org/wiki/1918_flu_pandemic (accessed 8 April 2018)

Chapter 5: We are already losing the arms race

15. Berg RD. Bacterial translocation from the gastrointestinal tract. *Advances in Experimental Medical Biology* 1999; 473: 11-30. (www.ncbi.nlm.nih.gov/pubmed/10659341)

16. Pond CM. *The Fats of Life*. Cambridge, UK: Cambridge University Press; 1998.

Chapter 6: Diet, micronutrients and sleep

17. In addition to our books see: http://drmyhill.co.uk/wiki/Fermentation_in_the_gut_and_CFS

18. Lim MM, Gerstner JR, Holtzman DM. Sleep–wake cycle and Alzheimer's disease: what do we know? *Neurodegener Dis Manag* 2014; 4(5): 351–362. (www.ncbi.nlm.nih.gov/pmc/articles/PMC4257134)

19. National Institutes of Health. How Sleep Clears the Brain. *NIH Research Matters* 28 October 2013 (www.nih.gov/news-events/nih-research-matters/how-sleep-clears-brain)

20. Kang P, de Bruin GS, Wang LH, Ward BA, Ances BM, Lim MM, Bucelli RC. Sleep pathology in Creutzfeldt-Jakob disease. *J Clin Sleep Med* 2016; 12(7): 1033–1039. (www.ncbi.nlm.nih.gov/pmc/articles/PMC4918986)

21. Jessen NA, Finnmann Munk AS, Lundgaard I, Nedergaard M. The Glymphatic System – A Beginner's Guide. *Neurochem Res* 2015; 40(12): 2583–2599. (www.ncbi.nlm.nih.gov/pmc/articles/PMC4636982)

22. Sánchez-Alavez M, Conti B, Moroncini G, Criado JR. Contributions of neuronal prion protein on sleep recovery and stress response following sleep deprivation. *Brain Research* 2007; 1158: 71–80. (www.ncbi.nlm.nih.gov/pmc/articles/PMC1994827)

23. Kam K, Duffy AM, Moretto J, LaFrancois JJ, Scharfman HE. Interictal spikes during sleep are an early defect in the Tg2576 mouse model of β-amyloid neuropathology. *Sci Rep* 2016; 6: 20119. (www.ncbi.nlm.nih.gov/pmc/articles/PMC4730189)

Chapter 7: Energy delivery mechanisms

24. Straub R. The brain and immune system prompt energy shortage in chronic inflammation and ageing. *Nature Reviews: Rheumatology* 2017; 13:743-751.

25. Úbeda F, Jansen VAA. The evolution of sex-specific virulence in infectious diseases. *Nature Communications* 2016; 7: article number 13849. (www.nature.com/articles/ncomms13849)

26. Anderson RM, May RM. Population biology of infectious diseases *Nature* 1979; 280(5721): 361-367. (www.ncbi.nlm.nih.gov/pubmed/460412?dopt=Abstract&holding=npg)

27. Baker R. Oxford University Lecture Notes – *Mathematical Modelling in Biology* https://courses.maths.ox.ac.uk/node/view_material/4272 (accessed 8 April 2018).

28. Foxman EF, Storer JA, Fitzgerald ME, Waski BR, et al. Temperature-dependent innate defense against the common cold virus limits viral replication at warm temperature in mouse airway cells. *Proceedings of the National Academy of Science USA* 2015; 112(3): 827-832. doi: 10.1073/pnas.1411030112

29. http://drmyhill.co.uk/wiki/Conducting_the_CFS_orchestra_–_how_to_put_yourself_in_charge

Chapter 8: The gut microbiome

30. www.columbia.edu/itc/mealac/pritchett/00litlinks/kautilya/book06.htm (English translation)

Chapter 9: Vitamin C

31. Smith LH. *Clinical Guide to the Use of Vitamin C. The Clinical Experiences of Frederick R. Klenner, M.D., abbreviated, summarised and annotated.* (www.seanet.com/~alexs/ascorbate/198x/smith-lh-clinical_guide_1988.htm – accessed 11 February 2018)
32. Klenner FR. Virus pneumonia and its treatment with vitamin C. *Southern Medicine and Surgery* 1948, 110(2): 36-38, 46. (www.mv.helsinki.fi/home/hemila/CP/Klenner_1948_ch.pdf)
33. Saul AW. Hidden in Plain Sight: The Pioneering Work of Frederick Robert Klenner, MD. *Journal of Orthomolecular Medicine* 2007; 22(1): 31-38. (www.doctoryourself.com/klennerbio.html – accessed 11 February 2018)
34. Cathcart RF. Vitamin C, titrating to bowel tolerance, anascorbia, and acute induced scurvy. *Medical Hypotheses* 1981; 7: 1359-1376. (https://vitamincfoundation.org/www.orthomed.com/titrate.htm – accessed 11 February 2018)
35. Levy TE. Vitamin C and sepsis – the genie is now out of the bottle. *Orthomolecular Medicine News Service* 24 May 2017.
36. Marik PE, Khangoora V, Rivera R, Hooper MH, Catravas J. Hydrocortisone, Vitamin C and Thiamine for the Treatment of Severe Sepsis and Septic Shock: A Retrospective Before-After Study. *Chest* 2017; 151(6): 1229-1238. doi: 10.1016/j.chest.2016.11.036. pubmed: 27940189

Chapter 10: Iodine – a great all-rounder

37. Selvaggi G, Monstrey S, Van Landuyt K, Hamdi M, Blondeel P. The role of iodine in antisepsis and wound management: a reappraisal. *Acta Chir Belg* 2003; 103(3): 241-247. pubmed 12914356
38. Derry D. Iodine: the Forgotten Weapon Against Influenza Viruses. *Thyroid Science*

2009; 4(9): R1-5. (www.thyroidscience.com/reviews/derry/Derry.flu.iodine.9.19.09.pdf)

39. The Cure Zone. Iodine is by far the best antibiotic. (www.curezone.org/blogs/fm.asp?i=1413057 – accessed 11 February 2018)

40. Abraham GE. for Volume 1 'Discovery to Essentiality' – (www.optimox.com/iodine-study-14)

41. Neuzil E. Jean Guillaume Auguste Lugol (1788-1851): his life and his works: a brief encounter, 150 years after his death. *Hist Sci Med* 2002; 36(4): 451-464. (www.ncbi.nlm.nih.gov/pubmed/12613445)

Chapter 11: Electromagnetic radiation – the good and the bad

42. Douwes F, Strasheim C. How I discovered hyperthermia for Lyme disease and why it works. *ProHealth* 7 February 2017. (www.prohealth.com/lyme/library/showarticle.cfm?libid=29931 – accessed 11 February 2018)

43. www.sciencemuseum.org.uk/broughttolife/techniques/heliotherapy (accessed 1 June 2018)

44. See http://www.mediclights.com for detail of this therapy and many pictures and videos too.

45. See http://www.medpagetoday.com/Neurology/GeneralNeurology/43985 (accessed 1 June 2018)

46. Cook Egg Using 2 Cell Phones (www.youtube.com/watch?v=oEkY8ALoJu4)

47. Cell Phone Radiation Pops Popcorn. www.youtube.com/watch?v=pqIZDIxJgXw

48. Pall ML. Electromagnetic fields act via activation of voltage-gated calcium channels to produce beneficial or adverse effects. *Journal of Cellular and Molecular Medicine* 2013; 17(8): 958–965. www.ncbi.nlm.nih.gov/pmc/articles/PMC3780531/

Chapter 12: Doctors, dentists and other foreign bodies

49. Wolf N. The silicone breast implant scandal. *The Guardian* 15 February 2012. (www.theguardian.com/commentisfree/cifamerica/2012/feb/15/silicone-breast-implant-scandal-naomi-wolf)

50. Francel TJ. Silicone-gel implant longevity (Abstract) In: *Proceedings of 67th*

Annual Scientific Meeting of the American Society of Plastic and Reconstructive Surgeons, 1998.

51. PetersWJ, Smith D, Lugowski S. Failure properties of 352 explanted silicone gel implants. *Canadian Journal of Plastic Surgery* 1996; 4(1):55-58.

52. Colaris MJL, de Boer M, van der Hulst RR, Cohen-Trevaert JW. Two hundred cases of ASIA syndrome following silicone implants: a comparative study of 30 years and a review of current literature. *Immunologic Research* 2017; 65(1): 120-128.

53. Leger M. Outbreak of *Mycobacterium chelonae* infection associated with tatoo ink. *New England Journal of Medicine* 2012; 367: 1020-1024.

Chapter 13: Herbals

54. Benzie IFF, Wachtel-Galor S. *Herbal Medicine: biomolecular and clinical aspects.* 2nd edition. CRC Press: 2011.You can access the full book online at this address: https://www.ncbi.nlm.nih.gov/books/NBK92771/

55. Disorides P. De Materia Medica. 50-70 AD. You can find free pdf files of all 5 volumes here – http://www.cancerlynx.com/dioscorides.html

56. Disorides P. De Materia Medica. 50-70 AD. www.cancerlynx.com/BOOKTHREEROOTS.PDF (Accessed 10 June 2018)

Chapter 14: Use your brain

57. Croft A. A lesson learnt: the rise and fall of Lariam and Halfan. *Journal of the Royal Society of Medicine* 2007; 100(4): 170–174. www.ncbi.nlm.nih.gov/pmc/articles/PMC1847738/

58. Biomonte S, et al. Morphine promotes tumor angiogenesis and increases breast cancer progression. *Biomed Research International* 2015; Article ID 161508.

58a. University of Chicago Medicine. Evidence mounts for link between opioids and cancer growth, 21 March 2012. http://www.uchospitals.edu/news/2012/20120321-opioid.html (Accessed 10 June 2018)

59. England C, Tomljenovic L. *Vaccination Policy and the UK Government: The Untold Truth*. CreateSpace Independent Publishing Platform, 2015.

60. www.telegraph.co.uk/news/health/news/5400079/One-in-every-64-children-could-have-autism-Cambridge-researchers-find.html).

61. Estimating the Prevalence of Autism Spectrum Conditions in Adults – extending the 2007 adult psychiatric morbidity survey. *NHS Digital* 31 January 2012. http://content.digital.nhs.uk/pubs/autism11 (accessed 3 April 2018)

62. Demicheli V, Rivetti A, Debalini MG, di Pietrantonj C. Vaccines for measles, mumps and rubella in children (Review). *Cochrane Library: Cochrane Database of Systematic Reviews* 2012; 2: CD004407. DOI: 10.1002/14651858.CD004407.pub3

Chapter 19: Measles, mumps, chicken pox and other such friendly immune programmers

63. Shah A, Coleman MP. Increasing incidence of childhood leukaemia: a controversy re-examined. *British Journal of Cancer* 2007; 97(7): 1009–1012. www.ncbi.nlm.nih.gov/pmc/articles/PMC2360402/

Chapter 21: Urinary tract infections (UTIs)

64. Berg RD. Bacterial translocation from the gastrointestinal tract. *Adv Exp Med Biol* 1999; 473: 11-30. www.ncbi.nlm.nih.gov/pubmed/10659341

65. Ettinger B, Pak CY, Citron JT, Thomas C, Adams-Huet B, Vangessel A. Potassium-magnesium citrate is an effective prophylaxis against recurrent calcium oxalate nephrolithiasis. *Journal of Urology* 1997; 158(6): 2069-2073. www.ncbi.nlm.nih.gov/pubmed/9366314

Chapter 22: Skin infections

66. https://forefrontdermatology.com/skin-fun-facts/ (Accessed 10 March 2018)

67. Cordain L, Lindeberg S, Hurtado M, Hill K, Eaton SB, Brand-Miller J. Acne vulgaris: a disease of Western civilization. *Archives of Dermatology* 2002; 138(12): 1584-1590. www.ncbi.nlm.nih.gov/pubmed/12472346

68. Dabre PD. Aluminium, antiperspirants and breast cancer. *Journal of Inorganic Biochemistry* 2005; 99(9): 1912-1919. www.ncbi.nlm.nih.gov/pubmed/16045991

Chapter 24: Dental infections and mouth ulcers

69. Peckham S, Awofeso N. Water Fluoridation: A Critical Review of the Physiological Effects of Ingested Fluoride as a Public Health Intervention. *The Scientific World Journal* Volume: 2014, Article ID: 293019. www.hindawi.com/journals/tswj/2014/293019/
70. Adler CJ et al. Sequencing ancient calcified dental plaque shows changes in oral microbiota with dietary shifts of the Neolithic and Industrial revolutions. *Nat Genet* 2013; 45(4): 450–455e1. www.ncbi.nlm.nih.gov/pmc/articles/PMC3996550/
71. http://news.nationalgeographic.com/news/2014/07/140716-sudan-sedge-toothbrush-teeth-archaeology-science/

Chapter 25: The fermenting gut

72. http://quotegardenterri.blogspot.co.uk/2016/07/james-lendall-basford.html (Accessed 10 June 2018)

Chapter 28: Principles of diagnosis of chronic 'stealth' infections

73. Burakgazi AZ. Lyme disease-induced polyradiculopathy mimicking amyotrophic lateral sclerosis. *International Journal of Neuroscience* 2014; 124(11): 859-862 (In the abstract.) www.tandfonline.com/doi/abs/10.3109/00207454.2013.879582

Chapter 31: Chronic infection of the gut

74. Jarosz M, Dzieniszewski J, Dabrowska-Ufniarz E, Wartanowicz M, Ziemlanski S, Reed PI. Effects of high dose vitamin C treatment on Helicobacter pylori infection and total vitamin C concentration in gastric juice. *European Journal of Cancer Prevention* 1998; 7(6): 449-454. www.ncbi.nlm.nih.gov/pubmed/9926292
75. Gui GP, Thomas PR, Tizard ML, Lake J, Sanderson JD, Hermon-Taylor J. Two-year-outcomes analysis of Crohn's disease treated with rifabutin and macrolide antibiotics. *Journal of Antimicrobial Chemotherapy* 1997; 39(3): 393–400. https://

academic.oup.com/jac/article/39/3/393/668334/Two-year-outcomes-analysis-of-Crohn-s-disease

76. Hoogkamp-Korstanje JA. Antibiotics in *Yersinia* enterocolitica infections. *Journal of Antimicrobial Chemotherapy* 1987; 20(1): 123-131. www.ncbi.nlm.nih.gov/pubmed/3497913

Chapter 32: Epstein Barr virus (EBV) and other herpes viruses

77. Draborg HA, Duus K, Houen G. Epstein-Barr virus in systemic autoimmune diseases. *Clinical Dev Immunology* 2013; 2013: 535738. www.ncbi.nlm.nih.gov/pmc/articles/PMC3766599/

78. Barker J. Epstein-Barr Virus: Its Connection to a Host of Different Diseases. www.cpmedical.net/newsletter/epstein-barr_virus_its_connection_to_a_host_of_different_diseases

79. Janegova A, Janega P, Rychly B, Kuracinova K, Babal P. The role of Epstein-Barr virus infection in the development of autoimmune thyroid diseases *Endokrynol Pol* 2015; 66(2): 132-136. doi: 10.5603/EP.2015.0020 www.ncbi.nlm.nih.gov/pubmed/25931043.

80. Bagert BA. Epstein-Barr virus in multiple sclerosis. *Current Neurology and Neuroscience Reports* 2009; 9(5): 405-410. www.ncbi.nlm.nih.gov/pubmed/19664371

81. Hjalgrim H, Friborf J, Melbye M. The epidemiology of EBV and its association with malignant disease. In: *Human Herpes Viruses: Biology, Therapy, and Immunoprophylaxis.* www.ncbi.nlm.nih.gov/books/NBK47424/

82. Konoshima T, Kikumai M, et al. Studies on inhibitors of skin tumor production. Inhibitory effects of flavonoids from *Scutellaria baicalensis* on Epstein-Barr virus activation and their anti-tumor-promoting activities. *Chem Pharm Bull* 1992; 40: 531-533. www.ncbi.nlm.nih.gov/pubmed/1318792

83. Lerner AM, Beqaj SH, Gill K, Edington J, Fitzgerald JT, Deeter RG. An update on the management of glandular fever (infectious mononucleosis) and its sequelae caused by Epstein–Barr virus (HHV-4): new and emerging treatment strategies. www.dovepress.com/an-update-on-the-management-of-glandular-fever-infectious-mononucleosi-peer-reviewed-article-VAAT

84. Li FY, Chaigne-Delaland B, Su H, Uzel G, Matthews H, Lenardo MJ. XMEN disease: a new primary immunodeficiency affecting Mg2+ regulation of immunity against Epstein-Barr virus. *Blood* 2014; 123(14): 2148-2152. doi: 10.1182/blood-2013-11-538686. Epub 2014 Feb 18. www.ncbi.nlm.nih.gov/pubmed/24550228

85. Epstein MA, Achong BG, Barr YM. Virus particles in cultured lymphoblasts from Burkitt's lymphoma. *Lancet* 1964; 1: 702–703.

Chapter 33: Lyme disease (*Borellia burgorferi*)

86. Horowitz RI. *How Can I Get Better? An action plan for treating resistant Lyme and chronic disease.* Tantor Media 2017.

Chapter 34: *Bartonella* and *Babesia*

87. Drancourt M, et al. *Bartonella Quintana* in a 4000-Year-Old Human Tooth. *Journal of Infectious Diseases* 2005; 191(4): 607-611. https://academic.oup.com/jid/article-lookup/doi/10.1086/427041

88. Nooten SS, Andrew NR, Hughes L. Potential impacts of climate change on insect communities: a transplant experiment. *PLoS One* 2014; 9(1): e85987. www.ncbi.nlm.nih.gov/pmc/articles/PMC3899090/

89. Hunfeld KP, Hildebrandt A, Gray JS. Babesiosis: Recent insights into an ancient disease. *International Journal for Parasitology* 2008; 38: 1219-1237 www.nslc.wustl.edu/courses/bio348/thach/2011/Babesiosis%20review.pdf

Chapter 35: *Mycoplasma* and *Chlamydia*

90. Haggerty CL, Taylor BD. *Mycoplasma genitalium*: An Emerging Cause of Pelvic Inflammatory Disease. *Infectious Diseases in Obstetrics and Gynecology* 2011; 2011 (2011). www.hindawi.com/journals/idog/2011/959816/

91. Larsen B, Hwang J. *Mycoplasma*, Ureaplasma, and Adverse Pregnancy Outcomes: A Fresh Look. *Infectious Diseases in Obstetrics and Gynecology* 2010; 2010 (2010). www.hindawi.com/journals/idog/2010/521921/

92. Miyashita N, et al. Clinical features of severe *Mycoplasma pneumoniae* pneumonia in adults admitted to an intensive care unit. *Journal of Medical Microbiology* 2007; 56: 1625–1629. www.microbiologyresearch.org/docserver/fulltext/jmm/56/12/1625.pdf

93. Ramirez AS, et al. Relationship between rheumatoid arthritis and *Mycoplasma pneumoniae*: a case–control study. *Rheumatology* 2005; 44(7): 912-914. https://academic.oup.com/rheumatology/article/44/7/912/1788375/Relationship-between-rheumatoid-arthritis-and

94. Johnson L, et al. *Mycoplasma*-like organisms in Hodgkin's disease. *Lancet* 1996; 347(9005): 901-902. www.thelancet.com/journals/lancet/article/PIIS0140-6736(96)91381-1/abstract

95. Sotgiu S, Pugliatti M, Rosati G, Deiana GA. Neurological disorders associated with *Mycoplasma pneumoniae* infection. *European Journal of Neurology* 2003; 10(2): 165-168. www.ncbi.nlm.nih.gov/pubmed/12603292

Chapter 37: Preventing antibiotic damage to the gut microbiome

96. Marik. Vitamin C and sepsis – The genie is now out of the bottle. *Orthomolecular Medicine News Service* May 24, 2017. http://orthomolecular.activehosted.com/index.php?action=social&chash=44f683a84163b3523afe57c2e008bc8c.66

Appendix

97. Moon S-E, Kim H-Y, Cha J-D. Synergistic effect between clove oil and its major compounds and antibiotics against oral bacteria. *Archives of Oral Biology* 2011; 56(9): 907-916.

Glossary

98. MacDonald A. *Alzheimer Borreliosis – My journal articles*. https://alzheimerborreliosis.net/research/ (accessed 25 April 2018).

Glossary

Amyloid – see Biofilm.

Autoimmunity – Autoimmunity occurs when the immune system has made a mistake. The immune system has a difficult job to do, because it has to distinguish between molecules which are dangerous to the body and molecules which are safe. Sometimes it gets its wires crossed and starts making antibodies against molecules which are 'safe'. For some people this results in allergies, which is a useless inflammation against 'safe' foreign molecules. For others this results in autoimmunity, which is a useless inflammation against the body's own molecules. These are acquired problems – we know that because they become much more common with age. It is likely we are seeing more autoimmunity because of Western lifestyles, diets and pollution. Chemicals, especially heavy metals, get stuck onto cells and change their 'appearance' to the immune system and thereby switch on inappropriate reactions. See my website (http://drmyhill.co.uk/ wiki/Autoimmune_diseases_-_the_environmental_approach_to_treating) for more information.

Bacterial allergy – See Viral allergy.

Biofilm – Biofilm is a barrier which microbes 'throw up' to hide themselves away from the body's natural defences. Examples of biofilm include dental plaque (*Streptococcus mutans*, the microbe responsible for dental decay, hides here), the coated tongue (microbes typically causing halitosis may hide here), gut mucopolysaccharide, fibrin

233

clots, amyloid (plaques form in the brain and are associated with Alzheimer's disease) and other such possibilities. Indeed, Dr Alan MacDonald has shown that in Lyme disease, *Borrelia* conceal themselves in amyloid.[98] Amyloid has been known about for years and is associated with many chronic diseases but its reason for existing is unknown. However, if amyloid is indeed the shield behind which microbes hide, then this opens up very interesting avenues for treatment of any disease associated with amyloid – that is to say, it may be a marker for a chronic inflammation driven by infection.

Faecal bacteriotherapy – The idea of faecal bacteriotherapy is to replenish the gut with friendly microbes. This treatment is of established benefit in inflammatory bowel disease and *Clostridium difficile* infections. It is also used in the veterinary world to treat animals with a range of gut symptoms. The difficult bug to replace is bacteroides because this does not survive for more than a few minutes outside the human gut. One needs a healthy donor 'on hand' to replenish with fresh material. For further details please see my website (www.drmyhill.co.uk/wiki/Faecal_bacteriotherapy) and also for information about the Borody Home Infusion Protocol (www.drmyhill.co.uk/drmyhill/images/4/49/Home_Infusion_protocol.pdf).

Herxheimer effect/reaction – The idea here is that if one kills microbes in the gut or elsewhere, it is possible to get an allergic reaction to the breakdown materials from these microbes wherever they happen to end up. In addition, the products released during the death of micro-organisms are endotoxin-like and so one also may experience a toxic-like effect. My patients who start my supplement and dietary regime often feel worse before they feel better; there are many reasons for this and perhaps the term Herxheimer is over-used to account for any such 'worsening' reactions – please see my website (www.drmyhill.co.uk/wiki/Getting_worse_on_the_regime_of_Stone_Age_diet_and_micronutrient_supplements_when_these_interventions_should_make_you_better#Herxheimer_reactions)

Inflammation – Inflammation is an essential part of our survival package. From an evolutionary perspective, the biggest killer of Homo sapiens (apart from Homo sapiens) has been infection, with cholera claiming a third of all deaths, ever. The body has to be alert to the possibility of any infection, to all of which it responds with inflammation. However, inflammation is metabolically expensive and inherently destructive. It has to be, in order to kill infections by bacteria, viruses, parasites or whatever. For example, part of the immune defence involves a 'scorched earth' policy – tissue immediately around an area of infection is destroyed so there is nothing for the invader to parasitise. The mechanism by which the immune system kills these infections is by firing free radicals at them. However, if it fires too many free radicals, then this 'friendly fire' will damage the body itself. Therefore, for inflammation to be effective it must be switched on, targeted, localised and then switched off. This entails extremely complex immune responses; clearly, there is great potential for things to go wrong. Inflammation is also involved in the healing process. Where there is damage by trauma, there will be dead cells. Inflammation is necessary to clear away these dead cells and lay down new tissues. Inflammation is characterised by heat and redness (heat alone is antiseptic), combined with swelling, pain and loss of function, which immobilises the area being attacked by the immune system. This is necessary because physical movement will tend to massage the infection to other sites. If one looks at life from the point of view of the immune system, it has a very difficult balancing act to manage. Too little reaction and we die from infection; too much reaction is metabolically expensive and damaging. If switched on inappropriately, the immune system has the power to kill us within seconds, an example of this being anaphylaxis. The NO/ONOO cycle is of importance here. This is a self-perpetuating pro-inflammatory cycle described by Professor Martin Pall. It is a central part of all processes involving inflammation. I think of it as a fire which is driven by many possible factors, including poor micronutrient and antioxidant status, toxic stress and immune activation (infections, autoimmunity and allergy). It perpetuates many vicious cycles – for example, poor mitochondrial function results in excessive free radicals being produced which, if not mopped up by anti-oxidants, further damage and inhibit mitochondrial function. The No-Oh-No cycle (appropriately named!) seems to have a momentum of its own, and once fired up it needs all possible interventions to damp the blaze.

Inflammatory markers – If the immune system is busy in the bloodstream, then inflammatory markers are raised and can be measured. The three most commonly used are erythrocyte sedimentation rate (ESR), plasma viscosity and a C-reactive protein. Raised inflammatory markers do not tell us the cause of the inflammation, simply that something is wrong. Raised inflammatory markers should always be taken seriously and properly investigated (see our second book *Sustainable Medicine* for more detail).

Ketoacidosis – Diabetic ketoacidosis is a potentially life-threatening complication caused by a lack of insulin in the body. This may occur if the body is unable to use blood sugar (glucose) as a source of fuel. Instead, the body breaks down fat as an alternative source of fuel. In ketosis, this breaking down of fat is desirable but because of the severity of the situation in diabetic ketoacidosis, this can lead to a dangerously high build-up of ketones.

Keto-adapted – A person who is 'keto-adapted' has made the switch from burning sugar and carbohydrates as a source of fuel to burning fats and fibre. One can test for this by testing for the presence of ketones in the blood or urine, although once fully keto-adapted, ketones may not show up in urine tests as the metabolism becomes more efficient. When keto-adapted, one's blood sugar level can run as low as 1 pmol/l without symptoms arising. See my website (www.drmyhill.co.uk/wiki/Ketogenic_diet_-_the_ practical_details) for further details of monitoring ketone levels and for the full story, please see our books *The PK Cookbook – go paleo-ketogenic and get the best of both worlds* and *Prevent and Cure Diabetes – delicious diets not dangerous drugs.*

Ketosis – Ketosis is a metabolic state where the majority of the body's energy supply is derived from ketone bodies in the blood. This is in contrast with a state of glycolysis where blood glucose provides the majority of the energy supply.

PK/paleo-ketogenic diet – The PK diet is a *combination* of the paleo diet (that which humans evolved into eating over a period of 2.5 million years) and the ketogenic diet.
- The paleo diet – Of course, in Paleolithic, pre-agricultural times there was no single diet – local conditions would have dictated what could be foraged and hunted. The constant factor would have been that no foods were cultivated. However, at the present time we use 'paleo diet' to denote one that consists of natural, unprocessed foods and rejects grains and dairy. The diet would have varied through the year with meat and fish being staples and with brief windows of time in autumn when natural harvests became available.
- The ketogenic diet – The body is remarkably adept at obtaining its fuels from a variety of foods.

Carbohydrates are not essential foods – we can survive without them. The fuel which actually enters our mitochondria (the power houses of all our cells) is acetate. One can get to acetate from fat via ketones and from fermenting vegetable fibre in the gut via short-chain fatty acids as well as from carbohydrates and proteins via glucose. The ketogenic diet is one that results in the metabolic state whereby the majority of the body's energy is derived from ketone bodies in the blood – the state of 'ketosis'. This is in contrast to the state of glycolysis where blood glucose provides the majority of the energy supply. For the full story, please see our books *The PK Cookbook – go paleo-ketogenic and get the best of both worlds* and *Prevent and Cure Diabetes – delicious diets not dangerous drugs.*

Viral allergy – The body can be sensitised and become allergic to anything. For example, I see many cases of allergic muscles where the body has become sensitised to food antigens. For example, tearing or bruising a muscle means that it comes in direct contact with blood, which may be carrying food antigens. I suspect the allergy is switched on at that time and the pain which follows the muscle damage, and which persists in the long term, is misattributed to damage, when actually it is sensitisation. So, a torn muscle in the back from, say, lifting a heavy load, could sensitise to, say, dairy products, and it is the consumption of dairy subsequently which keeps the problem on the boil. Allergic cystitis is another such example of sensitisation – microbes in the gut are miniscule compared with human cells and all too easily spill over into the bloodstream. They are excreted in urine and, indeed, normal human urine can contain up to 10,000 microbes per millilitre (ml) before it is declared to be infected. This is very confusing for women with allergic cystitis (and possibly men with prostatitis); they sensitise to these microbes and get all the symptoms of inflammation (pain, frequency and urgency, and sometimes even blood in the urine) when the bacterial counts in their urine are less than 10,000 microbes per ml. I think of this as **bacterial allergy**; it also responds to antibiotics because these greatly reduce the allergic load. So, in the same way, people may develop viral allergy – where the body becomes sensitised to a virus.

Postscript

Western medicine has lost its way. Doctors no longer look for the underlying causes of disease, a process which used to be called diagnosis, but rather seek a 'quick fix' response that will see the patient out of their surgery door in under ten minutes. This quick fix response usually comprises the prescribing of symptom-suppressing medications. Doctors have become the puppets of Big Pharma, dishing out drugs and working to a 'checklist' culture which is directed at the symptom, rather than the patient. Patients are seen as a collection of walking symptoms, rather than as people, each with a highly individual set of circumstances. Worse than this, not only do these prescription drugs do nothing to address the root causes of illness, but often they accelerate the underlying pathology and so drug prescribing snowballs. This leads to a vicious spiral of increasing drug costs, coupled with worsening pathologies for individual patients, whilst at the same time there is an increasing number of new, and chronic, patients, because their illnesses are never properly addressed at the root cause. It is no wonder that the National Health Service in the UK is being overwhelmed. The result is that millions suffer a painful, premature, and often lingering, death from diseases which are completely avoidable and reversible.

The time has come for patients to be empowered to take back control of their own health. To achieve this empowerment, they need:

1. The knowledge to work out why they have symptoms and disease.
2. Direct access to all relevant medical tests.
3. Direct access to knowledgeable health practitioners who can further advise and guide patients, together with direct access to safe and effective remedies.

None of this is beyond patients, who are always highly motivated to be well again and who always know their bodies better than anyone else. It is time to break down the artificial barriers that have been placed between patients and the direct access to medical knowledge, tests and experts that they so deserve.

This three-stage process of patient emancipation is addressed in the following ways:

1. The knowledge can be found in these five books:

a) *Sustainable Medicine*: This is the starting point for treating all symptoms and diseases. It explains why we have symptoms, such as fatigue and pain, and how we can work out the mechanisms of such symptoms and which are the appropriate medical tests to diagnose these mechanisms. Most importantly, *Sustainable Medicine* identifies the 'tools of the trade' to effect a cure. These tools include diets, nutritional supplements and natural remedies. These tools are sustainable because they reverse disease-mechanisms rather than escalate them.

b) *Prevent and Cure Diabetes – delicious diets not dangerous drugs*: All medical therapies should start with diet. Modern Western diets are driving our modern epidemics of diabetes, heart disease, cancer and dementia; this process is called metabolic syndrome. *Prevent and Cure Diabetes* explains in detail why and how we have arrived at a situation where the *real* weapons of mass destruction can be found in our kitchens. Importantly, it describes the vital steps every one of us can make to reverse this situation so that life can be lived to its full potential.

c) *Diagnosis and Treatment of Chronic Fatigue Syndrome and Myalgic Encephalitis – it's mitochondria, not hypochondria*: This book further explores the commonest symptom which people complain of – namely, fatigue – together with its pathological end result when this symptom is ignored. This is my [Dr Myhill's] life's work, having spent over 35 years in clinical practice, many months of academic research and the co-authoring of three scientific papers, all directed at solving this jigsaw puzzle of an illness. This book has application not just for the severely fatigued patient but also for the athlete looking for peak performance and for anyone wishing to increase their energy levels.

d) *The PK Cookbook – go Paleo-Ketogenic and get the best of both worlds*: This gives us the *how* of the PK diet while *Prevent and Cure Diabetes* gives us the *why*. This is the starting point for preventing and treating modern Western diseases, including diabetes, arterial disease, dementia and cancer. Dietary changes are always the most difficult, but also the most important, intervention. This book is based on my [Dr Myhill's] first-hand experience and research on developing a PK diet that is sustainable in the long term. Perhaps the most important feature of this diet is the PK bread – this has helped more people stick to this diet than all else! Secondly, it introduces PK salt (named 'Sunshine salt' because it is rich in vitamin D). This salt is comprised of all essential minerals (plus vitamins D and B12) in physiological amounts within a sea salt. This more than compensates for the mineral deficiencies that are ubiquitously present in all foods from Western agricultural systems. It is an essential and delicious addition to all modern Western diets.

e) *The Infection Game – life is an arms race*: This tells us why modern life is an arms race and which infections are driving Western diseases. It also details why we are losing this arms race and the clinical signs and symptoms that demonstrate this. Then comes the good news. There are chapters detailing the general approach to fighting infections and then also specific measures for specific infections, including EBV (glandular fever, 'mono'), Lyme disease, *Bartonella* and others. How to diagnose these infections is also covered and there are special sections on how to treat acute infections and also how to protect your microbiome. The vast majority of the approaches in this book are natural, including many herbal preparations, and can be done by the reader completely on their own, with no need to involve doctors. Prescription medications are reserved only for intransigent cases. Finally, you will learn about the unique 'groundhog' protocol for promoting and maintaining good health.

2. Access to medical tests

Many of these can be accessed directly through:
* www.bloodtestsdirect.co.uk/ where blood tests can be accessed directly without a doctor's request. Many can be done on fingerdrop samples of blood.

- www.arminlabs.com/en – blood tests can be accessed directly without the need for a referral from a doctor or health practitioner.
- www.biolab.co.uk/ – needs referral from a health practitioner – see NHW below.
- www.gdx.net/uk/ – Genova labs for stool, urine and saliva testing – needs referral from a health practitioner – see NHW below.

Tests include blood, urine, stool and saliva samples. Many blood tests can be carried out at home on a finger-drop sample of blood, without the need for a nurse or doctor to be involved at all.

3. Direct access to knowledgeable practitioners who can further advise and guide patients

Natural Health Worldwide is a website where any knowledgeable practitioner (medical doctor, qualified health professional or experienced patient) can offer their opinion to any patient. This opinion may be free, or for a fee, by telephone, email, Skype or Facetime. The practitioner needs no premises or support staff since bookings and payments are made online. Patients give feedback to that practitioner's Reputation page and star ratings evolve. See www.naturalhealthworldwide.com

Index